KU-315-933

thefacts

Lung cancer

EAST SUSSEX COUNTY COUNCIL
WITHDRAWN
-9 AUG 2024

04262737

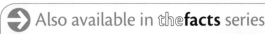# Also available in the**facts** series

the**facts**

Lung cancer

THIRD EDITION

STEPHEN FALK AND CHRIS WILLIAMS

Bristol Haematology and
Oncology Centre Bristol, UK

OXFORD
UNIVERSITY PRESS

OXFORD

UNIVERSITY PRESS

Great Clarendon Street, Oxford OX2 6DP

Oxford University Press is a department of the University of Oxford.
It furthers the University's objective of excellence in research, scholarship,
and education by publishing worldwide in

Oxford New York

Auckland Cape Town Dar es Salaam Hong Kong Karachi
Kuala Lumpur Madrid Melbourne Mexico City Nairobi
New Delhi Shanghai Taipei Toronto

With offices in

Argentina Austria Brazil Chile Czech Republic France Greece
Guatemala Hungary Italy Japan Poland Portugal Singapore
South Korea Switzerland Thailand Turkey Ukraine Vietnam

Oxford is a registered trade mark of Oxford University Press
in the UK and in certain other countries

Published in the United States
by Oxford University Press Inc., New York

© Oxford University Press 2010

The moral rights of the authors have been asserted
Database right Oxford University Press (maker)

First edition published 1984
Third edition published 2010

All rights reserved. No part of this publication may be reproduced,
stored in a retrieval system, or transmitted, in any form or by any means,
without the prior permission in writing of Oxford University Press,
or as expressly permitted by law, or under terms agreed with the appropriate
reprographics rights organization. Enquiries concerning reproduction
outside the scope of the above should be sent to the Rights Department,
Oxford University Press, at the address above

You must not circulate this book in any other binding or cover
and you must impose this same condition on any acquirer

British Library Cataloguing in Publication Data

Data available

Library of Congress Cataloging in Publication Data
Falk, Stephen A., 1945-
  Lung cancer / Stephen Falk and Chris Williams
    p. cm. — (Thefacts)
  Includes index.
  ISBN 978–0–19–956933–5
  1. Lungs Popular works.—Cancer I. Williams, C. J. (Christopher John
Hacon) II. Title.
  RC280.L8F27 2009
  616.99'424—dc22

                                                      2009028039
Typeset in Plantin
by Cepha Imaging Pvt. Ltd., Bangalore, India
Printed in Great Britain by Ashford Colour Press Ltd., Gosport, Hampshire

ISBN 978–0–19–956933–5

10 9 8 7 6 5 4 3 2 1

Whilst every effort has been made to ensure that the contents of this book are as complete, accurate
and up-to-date as possible at the date of writing, Oxford University Press is not able to give any
guarantee or assurance that such is the case. Readers are urged to take appropriately qualified
medical advice in all cases. The information in this book is intended to be useful to the general
reader, but should not be used as a means of self-diagnosis or for the prescription of medication.

Preface

Lung cancer is the commonest cancer in the Western world. The disease itself, and its effects on patients' families, thus afflicts thousands of us each year. The aim of this book is to give, in a clear and simple way, quite detailed information about all aspects of this type of cancer, with a stress on the practical side of its treatment. The first edition of this book was published in 1984 and this third edition has now has been completely revised. In the last 25 years there has been a remarkable decline in smoking habits. Changes in medical practice have delivered much better treatments and more patients are now undergoing treatment. This edition includes additional chapters asking the important questions as to what we can do to help ourselves, and explaining how the organization and delivery of National Health Service cancer care has improved.

Despite these improvements, lung cancer remains a scourge worldwide, with a poor outlook that is clearly related to smoking habits. Improving treatments and care will not replace, but reinforce the need for concerted worldwide tobacco control.

Stephen Falk

Chris Williams

Contents

Part 1

About lung cancer

1

What is lung cancer?

> ## → Key points
>
> ◆ Lung cancer is the most common cancer in the Western world.
> ◆ Cancer is defined as an abnormal growth of cells which tend to divide and grow in an uncontrolled way and, in some cases, to metastasize (spread).
> ◆ Treatment is determined by which of the two commonest types of lung cancer is present: small cell lung cancer or non-small cell lung cancer.

Introduction

Lung cancer is the most common cancer in the Western world. The disease itself, and its effects on patients' families, afflicts thousands of us each year. The aim of this book is to give, in a clear and simple way, quite detailed information about all aspects of this type of cancer, with a stress on the practical side of its treatment.

Before we can answer the question 'What is lung cancer?' we need to know what cancer itself is. The body is made up of millions of individual cells, most of which are capable of dividing and reproducing themselves so that the body can grow and, if injured, repair itself. The division of cells to form new cells is carefully controlled in the normal body, much as a car's speed is controlled by the brake and accelerator, so that extra, unwanted cells are not produced. A cut, for instance, will heal because the cells in the skin respond to a signal telling them to divide to form new cells, which fill in the injured area. However, as soon as the skin has healed, the cells appear to respond to another signal that tells them it is time to stop dividing. These control systems are remarkable in that faults in our genetic structure occur up to 15,000 times every day. Such faults are detected every day by the cells themselves or surrounding cells. The faulty cell will then either repair itself or more commonly self-destruct in a process known as apoptosis.

Rarely these mechanisms controlling cell divisions fail. Such a new cell may continue to divide, or simply not respond to the normal signals telling it to stop dividing. If this cell goes on dividing the new cells it produces are likely to lack the normal control mechanisms of cell division, and may carry on growing unchecked. Eventually these cells will form a cancer.

Under the microscope these abnormal cells pile up haphazardly where they start to grow, but they may also spread to other parts of the body by invading local tissues or through the blood vessels or lymphatic system (a network of fine vessels joining the lymph nodes; page 39).

The development of many cancers is, in reality, very much more complex and cells often undergo changes so that they are clearly abnormal but not yet cancerous (a premalignant stage) before they eventually become a malignant tumour. Many lung cancers go through this cycle and it is often possible to see these precancerous cells in the lining of the airways in the lung. The proportion of these abnormal cells that will eventually develop into cancer is about 30%. The fact that not all these abnormal cells actually develop into cancer gives scientists an opportunity to investigate those features that stop cancer developing and help deliver new preventative measures and treatments.

Characteristics by which cancer is defined

- ◆ Uncontrolled growth, which is unresponsive to the normal signals that tell cells when and when not to divide.
- ◆ Ability to invade local tissues.
- ◆ Ability to spread (metastasize) elsewhere in the body.

How does lung cancer occur?

Figures 1.1–1.5 show the sequence of events that takes place in the development of one particular type of lung cancer (squamous cancer; page 6).

1) There is inflammation of cells lining the airways into the lung, with loss of the lining cells (ciliated cells) that clear secretions from the airways, and overgrowth and piling up of deeper cells.

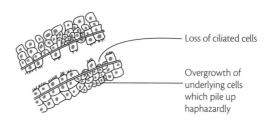

Loss of ciliated cells

Overgrowth of underlying cells which pile up haphazardly

2) The normal plump lining cells (columnar cells) of the airways change to a flatter type (squamous tells). This is referred to as metaplasia.

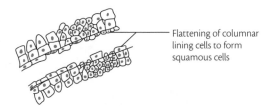

Flattening of columnar lining cells to form squamous cells

3) Increasingly abnormal metaplastic cells (now called dysplastic cells) appear. These changes are found in more than 90% of active smokers, in 6% of people who have stopped smoking for more than 5 years, and only in 1% of non-smokers. They are therefore reversible and do not mean that cancer is inevitable when dysplastic change has developed.

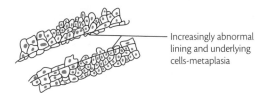

Increasingly abnormal lining and underlying cells-metaplasia

4) The next stage is called 'cancer *in situ*' (a small cancer that has not invaded or spread). This starts somewhere in the dysplastic area and may be several centimetres long and occupy the width of the lining of the airway. Cancer *in situ* is seen in the lungs of 1 in 20 heavy smokers.

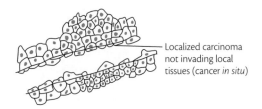

Localized carcinoma not invading local tissues (cancer *in situ*)

5) The small cancer *in situ* may then turn into an invasive cancer. The events that trigger the change from cancer *in situ* to a malignant tumour are not known. When the tumour starts to invade the nearby lung, lymph nodes, and other parts of the body it is regarded as a malignant lung cancer.

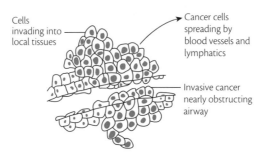

Types of lung cancer

Lung cancer is not one disease. Several kinds of cancer can develop in the lungs (Table 1.1) and each can be recognized by its appearance when looked at through a microscope. Each type tends to behave in a different manner and there is evidence that they may be caused in different ways. Although these differences are important for our future understanding of the disease they are not, at present, of much help to doctors when they are deciding on treatment. Because of this, the common lung cancers have been divided into two major groups for the purposes of choosing treatment (Table 1.1): small cell and non-small cell lung cancer.

Table 1.1 Main types of lung cancer

Type of cancer	Estimated incidence (%)
Non-small cell carcinoma	
Squamous carcinoma	35
Adenocarcinoma	27
Large cell carcinoma	10
Unclassified/undifferentiated	8
Small cell carcinoma	20

Mesothelioma, a tumour of the lining around the lungs (the pleura), differs greatly from these common lung cancers and is treated in a different way. It forms a third group of cancer affecting the lungs. There are also several rare types of cancer that can start in the lungs; these are discussed briefly in Chapter 9.

Many tumours that develop in other parts of the body may spread to the lungs; these should not be regarded as lung cancers but as secondary tumours in the lung. These tumours are treated not as lung cancer, but as the original tumour; they are not discussed further in this book.

Characteristics of the main types of lung cancer

Cancers types remain classified principally by their appearance under the light microscope using simple stains.

1. Squamous lung cancer

- This is the most common kind of lung cancer.
- It is called squamous carcinom a because its cells resemble a type of flat-surfaced cell called a squamous cell.
- The tumour cells produce keratin, a substance normally found in skin and hair.
- It is very much more common in smokers.
- It develops in the major airways (the large bronchi; Figure 5.2, page 37), and spreads by invading the local tissues, from where it spreads to lymph nodes and into the bloodstream.
- Extensive premalignant or dysplastic changes often accompany this tumour.

2. Adenocarcinoma

- This tumour is derived from glandular tissue.
- Adenocarcinomas usually develop beneath the lining (mucosa) of the airways.
- Many start in the periphery of the lung rather than in the centre of the chest.
- Smoking does not seem to predispose to the same extent as other types of lung cancer, but its rising incidence raises the possibility that filtering cigarettes has increased the risk.
- The tumour spreads in the airways and to lymph nodes, and eventually in the blood. Bronchoalveolar carcinoma is an unusual tumour arising from the lung tissue itself. There is often widespread involvement in both lungs. It is probably a special type of adenocarcinoma.

3. **Large cell carcinoma**

◆ These tumours show no attempt to form recognizable structures, like glands.

◆ They are usually found in smokers and may develop in the central or peripheral part of the lungs.

◆ They spread within the airways, to the lymph glands, and by the bloodstream.

4. **Small cell carcinoma**

◆ The cells of this tumour are small and fragile.

◆ Some are called 'oat cell', because of their similarity to oat grains.

◆ These cancers grow and spread rapidly through the bloodstream to other organs.

◆ They nearly always develop in smokers, usually in the central part of the lung.

◆ These tumours are thought to develop from a special type of cell concerned with making chemical messengers (hormones).

5. **Carcinoid**

◆ This is a rare type of lung cancer that also develops from the special hormone-producing cells.

◆ It has a much less malignant course than small cell lung cancer.

◆ It characteristically affects young people.

6. **Mesothelioma**

◆ This is a tumour of the lining or membrane (pleura) surrounding the lung and separating it from the chest wall (Figure 5.2, page 37).

◆ This tumour is typically associated with exposure to asbestos many years previously.

◆ It may also develop in the lining of the abdominal cavity—the peritoneum.

◆ Mesothelioma frequently causes fluid to accumulate between the lung and chest wall (a pleural effusion).

◆ They can be difficult to diagnose and to distinguish from other cancers that have spread from other parts of the body.

Tumour grade

This is a measure of the degree of normality of the individual tumour cells and of structures that they form when observed with a microscope. For instance, an adenocarcinoma that forms easily recognized glands is said to be of a good grade, or well-differentiated. Poorly differentiated tumours have very abnormal-looking cells and few recognizable normal structures and, because of this, it can be difficult to tell between a poorly differentiated adenocarcinoma and a large cell tumour, for example.

Sometimes therefore it is not always easy to be sure what type of cancer is present following light microscopy alone. Given the importance of making the correct diagnosis, additional special tests will then be performed in the laboratory. For patients this can lead to further anxieties as it may take a few more days to make the correct diagnosis.

Special tests
Monoclonal antibodies

Antibodies are proteins produced in the body which have the ability to recognize specific structures on other cells or proteins. We are now able to make antibodies in the laboratory which can recognize any one particular structure; these are called monoclonal antibodies. By attaching a marker to the monoclonal antibody, it is possible to show, using microscopy or other techniques, whether the monoclonal antibody is sticking preferentially to tumour cells or not. Monoclonal antibodies can be used to differentiate between tumours that are derived from different tissues but which look very similar under the microscope. For instance, small cell lung cancer may sometimes look like the cells seen in a cancer of the lymph glands (non-Hodgkin lymphoma). The difference in treatment and prognosis of these two conditions is huge. Using a technique known as immunohistochemistry we can quickly and clearly tell whether the tumour was derived from a lymph gland or the lung since we have developed monoclonals specific for structures on lymphoma cells and lung cancers. For example, TTF1 is a commonly used marker for adenocarcinoma of the lung but does not stain lymphomas.

The future

Each patient's cancer is unique in its genetic make-up. This is called the molecular footprint. As our knowledge of the genetic structure of both normal and tumour cell advances it is likely that treatment for cancer will change markedly. In the future, each tumour will have its molecular footprint determined in the laboratory and new treatments will be individualized to that particular cancer.

2

Who gets lung cancer?

 Key points

- At least 90% of lung cancers are related to smoking.
- Historically some occupations and chemicals increase the risk.
- Why exactly some smokers get cancer whereas others do not is unknown.
- Lung cancer affects over 3000 non-smokers a year in the UK.

Geography

Cancer of the lung is historically thought of as a disease of well-developed, affluent countries such as in the Western world. However, as the developing world becomes richer the incidence there is rising rapidly, associated directly with changes in cigarette consumption. Figure 2.1 shows changes in death rates from lung cancer in different countries associated with changes in smoking patterns. Worldwide around 1.3 billion people currently smoke cigarettes or other tobacco products. More men than women develop lung cancer, and it is a disease that becomes more common as we become more elderly with an average age of onset in the mid-70s.

The increase in the incidence of death from lung cancer since 1900 has been phenomenal; indeed, lung cancer was regarded as very rare until this century. Now lung cancer is the most common cancer in the world with 1.3 million people diagnosed in 2002. Worldwide, the highest rates of lung cancer in men are in Central and Eastern Europe and North America, and for women in North America. In the UK the rate of lung cancer peaked for men in the late 1970s, but since then has decreased by more than 40%. This reflects the decline in smoking rates in men after the Second World War. For women, lung cancer rates increased slowly until the late 1980s and have since stabilized.

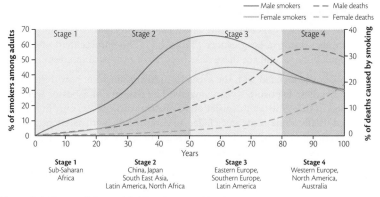

Figure 2.1 Stages of the worldwide tobacco epidemic.

Source: from Cancer Research UK, with permission, http://info.cancerresearchuk.org/cancerstats/types/lung/smoking/, accessed March 2009.

Lifestyle

> **Some statistics about lung cancer**
> - On average a smoker will die 10 years younger than a non-smoker.
> - Lung cancer is the cause of death in nearly 1 in 10 people who die in their 60s in industrialized societies.
> - 38,000 people in the UK die from lung cancer each year. Lung cancer is now the second most common cancer in men after prostate cancer, with more than 22,000 new cases diagnosed each year.
> - More than 16,000 women are diagnosed with lung cancer in the UK every year, making it the third most common cancer in women after breast and bowel cancer.

The next chapter discusses in more detail the possible causes of lung cancer but there are some factors that allow us to pick out those people at highest risk. The profile of someone at highest risk includes:

- living in an industrialized society;
- being a man;
- being a smoker;
- being aged 60 years or more;
- living in an urban environment.

Industry and chemicals

Exposure to certain cancer-causing chemicals or substances (carcinogens) at work can also result in lung cancer (Table 2.1). The enforcement of modern safety regulations should see these risks become of historical interest only.

The problems associated with the asbestos industry illustrate how difficult it is to avoid needless exposure to carcinogens. The dangers of asbestos were first recognised in the 1950s, but legislation to protect workers was only introduced in 1983. Initially some companies failed to comply fully with safety procedures and workers often ignored advice on precautions: and this happened despite our knowledge of some of the risks of asbestos.

Over time we will learn more about the cancer risks of various jobs and also the chemicals around us in the environment and how to reduce these risks (including banning some carcinogens). One of the main problems is the long time, known as the latent period, between exposure to the cancer-causing substance and the eventual development of a malignant tumour. Furthermore, often the carcinogen will increase the danger of a cancer developing rather than directly

Table 2.1 Jobs that historically have carried an increased risk of lung cancer[a]

Cancer-causing substance	Job
Arsenic	Oil refining, smelting, mining, using insecticides, tanning, working in the chemical industry
Chromium	Glassmaking, potting, acetylene and aniline manufacturing, bleaching, battery making
Iron oxide	Iron founding, iron ore mining, silver finishing, metal grinding and polishing
Asbestos	Asbestos milling and manufacture, working with insulation, shipyard working, brake and clutch repairing, asbestos mining
Petroleum products and oils	Working in contact with lubricating oils, paraffins or wax oils or coke and rubber
Coal tar and products	Working with asphalt, tar, and pitch, working in the coke-gas industry, working as a stoker, chimney-sweep, mining
Bis (chloromethyl) ether and mustard gas	Working in the chemical industry
Radiation	Working in the radiation industry, medicine, radiology

[a] Remember that not everyone in these industries is exposed to carcinogens. If you are concerned consult your company's doctor or your trade union.

cause it. This may be as long as 20 or more years and makes it difficult for workers and companies to take the risks seriously. Many people have and will die of cancer caused by a very short period of asbestos exposure 30 or 40 years earlier—the risks then only being appreciated when it is too late.

Anyone who may be exposed to carcinogens, such as asbestos, at work should try to stop smoking, as cigarettes seem to work together with the carcinogen and the two greatly increase the risk of lung cancer. Occasionally there may be a tendency for a family to be at high risk of developing cancer, and this may include cancers of the lung. However, only those family members who smoke or who are exposed to carcinogens are likely to get cancer.

No relationship between lung cancer and alcohol or drugs has been shown apart from smoking marijuana which is linked to the deep inhalation of tobacco associated with it. Air pollution has never been conclusively shown to cause cancer, although those who live in urban areas with more pollution seem to have a higher risk. Radon gas in the environment is increasingly recognized as an important but unavoidable risk factor.

What we do not know and are unable to predict is why some individuals who smoke very heavily get lung cancer whereas others do not.

3

What causes lung cancer?

 Key points

- The major cause of lung cancer is smoking.
- The chance of getting lung cancer is related to the total number of cigarettes consumed.
- Cigarette smoking can also result in other diseases often affecting the lungs and heart.
- On average smokers die 10 years younger than non-smokers.

Lung cancer is a disease of the twentieth century. Indeed, in 1912 a well-known US doctor wrote: 'primary cancers of the lung are among the rarest forms of the disease'. Medical students of that day hardly saw a single case during their training; unfortunately this is far from the case now. Lung cancer is now the most common tumour in the developed world. Any explanation of the cause of lung cancer must, therefore, take into account the huge increase, and latterly decrease, in the incidence of this cancer this century (Figures 3.1 and 3.2). The geographical distributions of the tumour must also be considered. These factors strongly suggest environmental causes and rule out genetic factors, because the genetic make-up of the population could not change so quickly. Lung cancer has been blamed on many factors and, although there are some who continue to believe otherwise, the close match to cigarette smoking trends shown in Figure 2.1 is inescapable.

Smoking

The habit of smoking, chewing, or taking tobacco as snuff has been common in Europe for more than 400 years, so why should there be a sudden increase in lung cancer deaths? Although tobacco has been used for a long time, it is only in the past hundred years that cigarette smoking has been commonplace, and only in the twentieth century that tobacco has become mild enough to be inhaled into the lungs. It is the inhalation of tobacco smoke deep into the lungs that causes lung cancer, and this is a relatively recent habit.

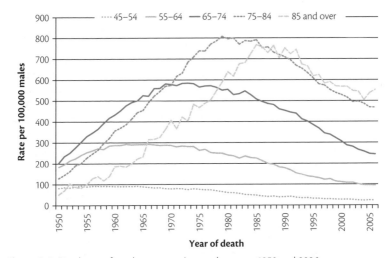

Figure 3.1 Death rates from lung cancer in men between 1950 and 2006.

Source: from Cancer Research UK, with permission, http://info.cancerresearchuk.org/cancerstats/types/lung/mortality/, accessed March 2009.

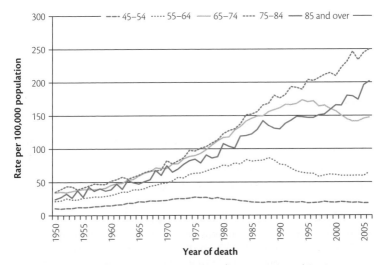

Figure 3.2 Death rates from lung cancer in women between 1950 and 2006.

Source: from Cancer Research UK, with permission, http://info.cancerresearchuk.org/cancerstats/types/lung/mortality/, accessed March 2009.

In the 1600s tobacco was usually smoked in pipes by men. It was the invention of cigarette-making machines in the latter part of the nineteenth century that made mass consumption of tobacco possible. Cigarette smoking as we know it really started during the Crimean War (1853–6), and the first major boost in tobacco sales came with the First World War. Cigarettes were lauded for their ability to induce tranquillity and to relieve depression, thirst, and hunger, and every effort was made to ensure that front-line troops received free cigarettes—they were even described by one General as being: 'as indispensable as the daily ration'.

Following the First World War cigarette sales fell, but intensive advertising and the handing out of free 'starter' packs ensured that more and more men, and then women, became smokers. By the 1930s the majority of the population in the UK were smokers and the trend towards increased smoking continued. At this time several reports linking smoking and deaths from lung cancer were published in Germany and the USA. However, the numbers of patients involved were relatively small and the evidence was ignored. The onset of the Second World War stopped further investigation of the risks of cigarette smoking and sales rose even further. In 1945 consumption peaked at an incredible 12 manufactured cigarettes per adult male per day. Advertising even continued in American medical journals, encouraging doctors with slogans such as: 'the thoughtful physician sends cigarettes to his friends and patients overseas'. Smoking was seen as socially desirable and few doctors had any qualms about its safety.

Investigation of the link between smoking and lung cancer

After the Second World War, research workers again started to examine the effects of smoking on health. Initially these studies reviewed the smoking habits of a group of patients with lung cancer and compared them with the smoking habits of a similar group of individuals not suffering from lung cancer (a retrospective survey called a case–control study).

Retrospective surveys

At least 30 retrospective investigations from 10 countries have shown that among patients with lung cancer there is a higher proportion of heavy smokers than in comparable control groups. Not only have all these studies shown the same association, but in general the results from different countries have been very similar.

The method of investigation used is to record answers to questions about smoking habits given by patients with lung cancer and to compare them with those given by matched individuals without the disease, usually patients in the same hospital. Despite scrupulous care in running such surveys, the results are always open to the criticism that an unknown bias may have affected the results.

Although much of the criticism of these early studies was successfully refuted, new studies in fit and healthy populations to find their risk of *developing* lung cancer according to their smoking habit were clearly needed. Such studies are called prospective surveys.

Prospective surveys

Doll and Hill, the researchers who started retrospective studies in the UK in the 1950s followed these with a prospective study in more than 40,000 male doctors. In the USA several groups of workers, including Hammond and Horn, and Dorn, started similar studies with even larger groups.

All of these prospective studies confirmed the results of the retrospective studies, and the results of the large prospective studies conducted so far (at least eight) are very similar. All show a steady increase in the number of deaths from lung cancer with increasing cigarette consumption. The increase in the number of deaths with the number of cigarettes smoked in three of the largest studies is shown in Figure 3.3. Although these studies have been criticized on the grounds that none of them was carried out on a strictly random sample of any population, their unanimous finding that the risk of death from lung cancer is closely associated with cigarette smoking, and to a smaller extent with other forms of smoking, is unchallenged. In addition, postmortem studies of the lungs of people who have died of diseases other than lung cancer have shown that precancerous changes in the lining of the airways, of a kind pathologists regard as predisposing to cancer (page 5), are common in smokers but seldom seen in non-smokers.

Prospective studies show that the risk of developing lung cancer increases with the number of cigarettes smoked (a dose–response effect; Figure 3.3), and

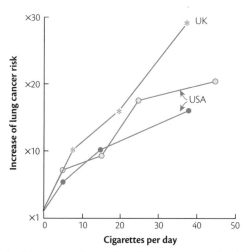

Figure 3.3 Relationship between the number of cigarettes smoked and the risk of death from lung cancer in three prospective studies.

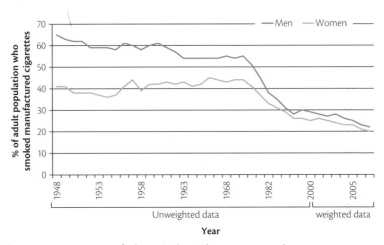

Figure 3.4 Consumption of tobacco in the UK between 1948 and 2007.
Source: from Cancer Research UK, with permission, http://info.cancerresearchuk.org/
cancerstats/types/lung/smoking/, accessed March 2009.

that the way in which an individual smokes influences the cancer risk. The risk of developing lung cancer is greater in those who inhale the cigarette smoke, who start early in life, who take more puffs on each cigarette, who keep the cigarette in the mouth between puffs, and who relight half-smoked cigarettes. In these studies men who switched to filter-tipped cigarettes during the previous 10 years were about 40% less likely to develop lung cancer than those who continued to smoke plain cigarettes. Smokers could be forgiven for believing that low-tar cigarettes deliver less tar to the smoker's lung. However, the actual tar exposure and hence health risk from smoking low-tar brands is likely to be the same as for conventional cigarettes.

This prospective and retrospective evidence thus links smoking and lung cancer deaths with the high incidence of smoking among patients with lung cancer. It also shows a clear dose–response effect and further implicates cigarette smoking by the changes in death rate related to subtle variations in the ways in which cigarettes are smoked and the type of cigarettes used. The parallel lines of deaths from lung cancer and cigarette consumption are compelling. After the Second World War there was a slight dip in consumption, but thereafter it remained at around 10 manufactured cigarettes per day until 1974, which marked the start of a steady and continuous decrease to 4.6 manufactured cigarettes per adult male per day by 1992 (Figure 3.4). The good news is that tobacco consumption is now falling quickly, but still around a fifth (22%) of the British population aged 16 and over smoke cigarettes, equating to about 9.5 million people in the UK. A further one million people smoke pipes/cigars.

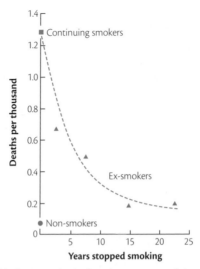

Figure 3.5 Relationship between deaths from lung cancer and time since stopping smoking cigarettes.

Doctors measure total tobacco use by pack-year. Pack-year is a term used to describe the number of cigarettes a person has smoked over time. One pack-year is defined as 20 manufactured cigarettes (one pack) smoked per day for one year. Smoking 1½ packs per day for 26 years equals 39 pack-years.

If cigarette smoking does cause lung cancer, a further powerful piece of evidence confirming this would be a reduction in the death rate from lung cancer of individuals stopping smoking.

Reduction of risk on stopping smoking

All studies have shown a marked reduction of risk of dying from lung cancer in those who have stopped smoking cigarettes compared with those who continue to smoke. This relative reduction is apparent within a few years of stopping. After about 10 years the ex-smoker's risk is only about one-quarter of that of the continuing smoker. The beneficial effect of stopping smoking on lung cancer is best shown in Doll and Hill's study of British doctors, in which more than 50% of the smokers stopped during the course of the 20-year study. Between 1954 and 1965 the death rate from lung cancer for these male doctors fell by a staggering 38%, while the rate for all men in the country (whose consumption of tobacco increased slightly) rose by 7%. When the mortality (death rate) of ex-smokers is looked at in relation to the number of years from stopping smoking, a clear benefit for stopping smoking is seen. Many cigarette smokers think that if they have smoked for 20 or more years it is too late to stop smoking

Some smoking statistics

- The highest rates of smoking are in the 20–24-year age group, with 32% of people this age recorded as smokers.

- The prevalence of smoking then declines with age, to 14% of people aged 60 years and older being smokers.

- Originally there was no difference between social class of smokers. Now, 29% of adults in manual occupations smoke compared to 19% of those in non-manual occupations.

- Smoking is a key contributory factor to health inequalities between socio-economic groups in the UK and accounts for a major part of the differences in life expectancy between manual and non-manual groups of workers.

- Smoking rates vary considerably between ethnic groups and between men and women within those groups. In men, smoking rates ranged from 20% (Indian) to 40% (Bangladeshi) compared with the national average of 24%. In women the rates ranged from 2% (Bangladeshi) to 26% (Irish) compared with the national average of 23% (Figure 3.6).

- In the UK, Scotland has the highest smoking prevalence rate at 27%, followed by Northern Ireland (26%), England (24%), and Wales (22%).

- Within the EU there is wide variation in smoking prevalence from around 18% in Sweden to 42% in Greece. The average for the 25 countries of the EU was 32%.

- While fewer than 1% of 11- and 12-year-old children smoke, by the age of 15 years, 1 in 5 (20%) children are regular smokers in England despite the fact that it is illegal to sell any tobacco product to under-18s.

- Since 1986, girls have had consistently higher rates of smoking than boys: in 2006, 24% of 15-year-old girls were regular smokers compared with 16% of boys.

- On average, regular child smokers smoke 42 cigarettes per week.

because they have already damaged their lungs, but Figure 3.5 shows that this is just not true.

Passive smoking

Non-smoking spouses of smokers have a small but definitely increased risk of developing lung cancer. Much of this information has come from a study of non-smoking wives of Japanese smokers, and it is thought that these women were inhaling the cigarette smoke of their spouse (so-called passive smoking). Someone who does not smoke but whose spouse smokes more than 20 cigarettes per day has twice the risk of lung cancer than if their spouse were a non-smoker. In addition, passive smoking also contributes to continuing the 'family circle' of smoking and there is much evidence of the harmful effects on children in 'smoking' households including respiratory disease, asthma attacks, cot deaths, and middle ear infections. This is why many countries have now banned smoking in public places. As well as removing the unpleasant (for non-smokers) effects of cigarette smoking, the risk of lung cancer for the population as a whole should reduce. This will be helped by emerging evidence that where bans have been enforced there has been rapid and sustained falls in overall tobacco consumption.

Other causes of lung cancer

Radon

The radioactive gas radon was first recognized to increase the risk of lung cancer in uranium miners. Radon can also be released from the ground into the foundations of some buildings and, if the buildings are well insulated, the gas may reach relatively high concentrations. Radon levels vary greatly from one part of the country to another and high levels are only found in certain locations, for example in the South West of England. It is an unavoidable risk but is probably the second commonest cause of lung cancer, accounting for up to 9% of cases.

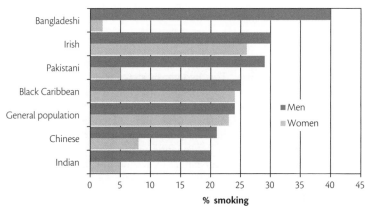

Figure 3.6 Self-reported cigarette smoking percentages by sex and minority ethnic group, persons aged 16 years and over, England, 2004.

Source: from Cancer Research UK, with permission, http://info.cancerresearchuk.org/cancerstats/types/lung/smoking/, accessed March 2009.

Air pollution

Air pollution, particularly smoke from fossil fuels, appears to increase the risk of lung cancer but its effect is small compared with that of cigarette smoking. As fossil fuel use falls, the evidence is now strongest for an increased risk of lung cancer caused by exposure to nitrogen oxides, particularly exposure to traffic fumes. It is difficult to estimate the effects of air pollution as those people exposed to air pollution, in industrialized urban areas for instance, are often the people also at risk from excessive smoking and from their jobs. Certain occupations (Table 2.1, page 12) that allow exposure to large quantities of herbicides and insecticides, asbestos dust, chromate, nickel, arsenic, radioactive materials, mustard gas, and the products of coal distillation in the gas industry may also have an increased risk of developing lung cancer, particularly if the exposed individuals are also smokers. However, the number of people at work in such occupations is relatively small and the greatly increased number of deaths from lung cancer cannot be explained by occupational exposure alone.

Diet

Japanese studies have shown that people deficient in vitamin A (found in green-yellow vegetables) have a higher risk of lung cancer. This vitamin has not been tested to see if supplements to the diet will reduce the risk of lung cancer, although many Western foods already have added vitamins added (breakfast cereals for example). The evidence for diet and the risk of lung cancer in Western populations remains uncertain. A diet rich in fruit and vegetables may be associated with a reduced risk of lung cancer, but the protective effect is probably limited to smokers.

Genetic factors

It has been suggested that the association between lung cancer and smoking is genetic rather than causal. This hypothesis states that the liability to lung cancer and the desire to smoke cigarettes are inherited genetically and are closely linked. In support of this hypothesis is evidence from studies of twins suggesting a genetic factor in smoking habits and differences between smokers and non-smokers in both physical and psychological characteristics. However, this hypothesis seems an unlikely explanation of the association between lung cancer and smoking because of the failure to account for the great increase in deaths from lung cancer this century.

As a genetically determined disease could not change its frequency in such a short time, advocates of this hypothesis can only explain the increase in lung cancer on the basis that other tumours or diseases were previously diagnosed mistakenly. However, this would not explain the earlier rise in the incidence of lung cancer in men, as changes in diagnostic accuracy would not be confined to one sex. The genetic trait theory also completely fails to account for the fall in the incidence of lung cancer deaths seen in those who stop smoking.

Genetic influences may, however, determine which smokers are likely to develop lung cancer. There is some evidence that cancers, including lung cancer, may be more common in certain families. Only a minority of smokers develop lung cancer and those who do so may have an inherited trait that makes them more susceptible to the cancer-causing factors in cigarette smoke. But even lung-cancer-prone individuals rarely develop the tumour unless they inhale a cancer-producing substance—which for most people is cigarette smoke.

However, a family history of lung cancer in a first-degree relative, i.e. mother, father, brother, or sister, results in a two-fold increased risk, independent of smoking. If both cancers are diagnosed before the age of 60 years, the risk ratio is almost five-fold. The association between family history and risk may be stronger in Black individuals than White.

Previous cancer treatment and lung cancer risk

Many young people are now surviving cancer and living long enough to develop a second or indeed even a third cancer. Treatment for Hodgkin's lymphoma increases lung cancer risk by 2.6–7-fold. Risk ratios are higher in smokers than non-smokers and for those treated with radiotherapy compared to chemotherapy alone. An increased risk of lung cancer has also been shown after treatment for non-Hodgkin's lymphoma, and up to 30 years after diagnosis with testicular cancer, which is largely linked to previous radiotherapy to the chest as part of the treatment.

Other factors and lung cancer risk

Significant increases in the risk of developing lung cancer have been reported in people with human immunodeficiency virus (HIV) and acquired immune deficiency syndrome (AIDS) even after accounting for smoking habits, although one study showed an association in men only.

People with antibodies to *Chlamydia pneumoniae* have a small increase in risk. *C. pneumoniae* is an infectious bacterium associated with a number of diseases including pneumonia. An increased risk of lung cancer has been shown in people with systemic lupus erythematosus (a rare autoimmune condition) and with Klinefelter syndrome (an inherited disorder), in both cases less than two-fold.

Other diseases related to cigarette smoking

Today, tobacco consumption is recognized as the UK's single greatest cause of preventable illness and early death, with more than 114,000 people dying each year from smoking-related diseases including cancers.

Other cancers

Although public awareness of the potential hazards of cigarette smoking is centred on lung cancer, this is only one of many diseases related to smoking. Other types of cancer are more frequent in smokers and a relationship similar to that shown in lung cancer exists. Around 90% of lung cancer cases are caused by tobacco smoking, and it is now agreed that tobacco smoking can also cause cancers of the following sites: upper aero-digestive tract (oral cavity, nasal cavity, nasal sinuses, pharynx, larynx, and oesophagus), pancreas, stomach, liver, lower urinary tract (renal pelvis and bladder), kidney, uterine cervix, and myeloid leu-kaemia. Overall tobacco smoking is estimated to be responsible for about 30% of cancer deaths in developed countries, i.e. 46,000 deaths in 2005 in the UK.

Diseases of the heart and blood vessels

Increased illness and death from diseases of the heart and blood vessels, despite public concentration on the risks of lung cancer, are more important effects of cigarette smoking than cancer (Table 3.1). Heart and blood vessel disease accounted for more than half the extra deaths in smokers in Doll's study of British doctors. When coronary heart disease is studied in detail, the incidence of deaths increases with the number of cigarettes smoked at all ages, although it is greatest in young people. In men under 45 years of age the death rate per 100,000 was 7 for non-smokers and 104 for those who smoked more than 25 cigarettes per day. Although the mechanism of the association is unknown, evidence suggests that the inhalation of carbon monoxide and nicotine may be contributory factors.

Early reports have suggested that the introduction of filter-tipped cigarettes (which probably reduce the incidence of lung cancer) may result in high blood levels of carbon monoxide and potentially increase the incidence of heart or cardiovascular disease.

The effect of smoking on lung cancer is reversible, and this is also true for car-diovascular disease. In the British doctors' study the death rate from coronary

Table 3.1 Excess deaths in male smokers by various causes (study of British doctors)

Cause of death	No. of extra (excess) deaths per 100,000 smokers per year
Lung cancer	94 (19%)
Chronic bronchitis and emphysema	47 (10%)
Coronary heart disease	152 (31%)
Other vascular diseases and strokes	100 (21%)
Other diseases	92 (19%)
Total	485 (100%)

heart disease in men under 65 years fell steadily throughout the study; in older men there was little change. When the death rate is studied by smoking habit and the time from stopping smoking it is found that for both light and heavy smokers it takes about 10–15 years for the risk from coronary heart disease to fall to that of non-smokers.

Bronchitis and emphysema

Chronic bronchitis and emphysema account for about 10% of the extra deaths caused by smoking. The incidence of bronchitis has been falling for the past 40–50 years and the most likely explanation for this is reduced air pollution, decreasing tar content in cigarettes, and improved treatment. However, bronchitis and emphysema are clearly related to cigarette smoking and tests of lung function show impairment, which is most marked in heavy smokers. The damage caused by smoking in this condition is mechanical and stopping smoking does not result in improved lung function, although the rate of deterioration is slowed.

Smoking in pregnancy

Pregnant women who smoke also put their unborn baby at risk: more still-births, preterm births, spontaneous abortions and small babies who die early are born to smokers than to non-smokers. The babies of women who smoke weigh on average 200 g (7 oz) less than those of non-smokers. Infants and children whose parents smoke are also more prone to chest infections.

Numerous other illnesses are related to smoking and the dangers of cigarette smoking are clearly not confined to an increased risk of lung cancer. As a consequence of tobacco-related illness, the average smoker lives for 10 years less than a non-smoker.

Smoking and lung cancer

- The risk of death from lung cancer is related to the number of cigarettes smoked and the age of starting, and is reduced by smoking filter-tipped cigarettes. There is a small but significant risk for non-smokers when they regularly inhale cigarette smoke (passive smoking).

- Giving up smoking reduces the risk of death from lung cancer compared to those who continue to smoke; after 15 years, the risk falls to a level similar to that for non-smokers. For those who do not stop smoking, filter-tipped low-tar cigarettes are a step in the right direction as long as consumption is not increased by smoking more of each cigarette or increasing the number of cigarettes smoked each day.

- ◆ The incidence of lung cancer is increased by exposure to certain chemicals used in industry.

- ◆ There may be a genetic predisposition to lung cancer, as not all heavy smokers develop cancer. However, individuals predisposed to lung cancer may only develop the tumour on exposure to carcinogens such as cigarette smoke.

- ◆ Smoking also increases the death rate from other diseases. Of these, by far the most important is cardiovascular disease (which causes over half the extra deaths due to smoking). Cigarette smoking is also linked to various other tumours, chronic bronchitis, and emphysema. The risk of cardiovascular disease is reduced by stopping smoking and is similar to that of non-smokers 10–15 years after stopping smoking.

Smoking is by far the single most important avoidable cause of ill health and death in the industrialized world.

4

Stopping smoking

> ## → Key points
>
> ◆ You have to decide that you want to stop smoking.
> ◆ Get all the help you need.
> ◆ Access the National Health Service (NHS) Stop Smoking Service.
> ◆ Encourage your friends and families to stop too.
> ◆ Reward yourself for being a non-smoker with the money you have saved.

A healthier lifestyle

We are constantly bombarded with information about our apparently unhealthy lifestyles with advice about the food we eat, quantity of alcohol we drink, and the amount of exercise we take. However, the reality is that for smokers, breaking this habit outweighs any other lifestyle change in prolonging length of life and improving health. It may sound as though it should be easy to give up smoking, but this is far from the case. Tobacco is a remarkably addictive drug. The most important first point—strength of will—comes from deciding for yourself that you want to stop, rather than just being pressured by your family and friends. If you do not believe there is sufficient reason to stop, it will be very difficult, if not impossible.

So, the first step is deciding if you really want to stop, and if so, why?

> ## The advantages of stopping smoking
>
> ◆ The risk to your health (see Chapter 3): there is an increased risk of lung cancer, heart disease, chronic bronchitis, other cancers, ulcers, and many other conditions. Although many smokers scoff at the thought, and try to pretend that it is scaremongering, the risks are deadly serious. Many life assurance companies now offer reduced premiums for non-smokers, and they only bet on certainties. On average those dying of diseases caused by smoking lose 10–15 years of their life.

- ◆ The cost: most smokers would have an extra £20–50 per week to spend.
- ◆ You will feel healthier and will be able to breathe more easily when you take exercise.
- ◆ You will smell fresher and won't have bad breath and stained teeth and fingers.
- ◆ You will have fewer colds and chest infections.
- ◆ Your children will be less likely to start smoking.
- ◆ You will reduce any risk of chest problems for the rest of your family.

To a non-smoker this list seems compelling; who would not prefer to save hundreds of pounds a year and have the chance of better health? Many smokers seem blind to the risks and would say that health is more important to them than wealth—even as they light up their next cigarette. You will have taken the first step in stopping smoking when you really believe that cigarettes are bad for you and that you will also gain positive advantages from stopping. You must believe that the advantages of stopping outweigh the discomforts. A good place to start is to ask yourself why you smoke and also why would you want to stop?

There are many ways of approaching the problem and no easy solutions. On pages 31–32 there is a list of organizations who may be able to help you to stop smoking. This may be by providing direct help in clinics that support people stopping smoking or by giving information. It is useful to see your GP, who may be able to help you personally or put you in touch with a local group. The NHS has sensibly targeted smoking cessation as an important public health measure. As a result it now provides a number of services to help including:

- ◆ **Stop smoking groups**—sessions run by health professionals for groups of smokers who want to stop. In the sessions you can find out more about ways to give up and share tips and experiences with others.
- ◆ **One-to-one counselling**—in many areas individual counselling is available to help you give up.
- ◆ **QUIT** is an independent charity with comprehensive written, web-based, and interactive advice.

Methods used to help smokers quit include:

- ◆ *Drug therapy*. Historically this consisted entirely of tranquillizers which are ineffective and best avoided.
- ◆ There are currently a number of tobacco substitutes available both on and off prescription.

◆ *Nicotine replacement therapy* (NRT) works differently to cigarettes. It does not contain toxic chemicals such as tar or carbon monoxide, and does not cause cancer. NRT is suitable for most people. NRT is available in many different preparations including gums, sprays, patches, tablets, lozenges, and inhalers. NRT has been shown to double your chances of successfully quitting.

◆ There are also two prescription drugs:

Bupropion hydrochloride (Zyban®) is a treatment which changes the way that your body responds to nicotine. You start taking Zyban 1–2 weeks before you quit and treatment usually lasts for a couple of months to help you through the withdrawal cravings.

Varenicline (Champix®) works by reducing your craving for a cigarette and by reducing the effects you feel if you do have a cigarette. You set a date to stop smoking, and start taking tablets 1 or 2 weeks before this date. Treatment normally lasts for 12 weeks. Being low in mood may be a symptom of nicotine withdrawal. Depression, rarely including suicidal ideation (thinking about committing suicide) and suicide attempt, has been reported in people trying to stop smoking. These symptoms have also been seen while attempting to quit smoking with varenicline.

◆ *Hypnosis*. Although individual practitioners have claimed high success rates, there have been no properly controlled trials testing the effectiveness of hypnosis. It seems to suit some smokers, although this may depend on the skill of the therapist and the motivation of the smoker, which could be related to the amount of money the client pays for the treatment.

◆ *Exercise*. Doing exercise while stopping smoking can increase your chances of quitting successfully.

◆ *Acupuncture*. Once again, no studies have adequately tested the effectiveness of acupuncture. Some smokers seem to find it helpful.

◆ *Aversion therapy*. This is usually a form of oversmoking or rapid smoking designed to make smoking so unpleasant that the smoker cannot tolerate any more. There is little evidence that it works for very long, although it may well take away the desire to smoke for a short period.

◆ *Group therapy*. You could join a 'stop smoking support group'. This can help you feel less alone, find new coping skills, and motivate you to stick to treatment plans, and share your positive experiences of stopping smoking.

◆ *Placebo*. Some antismoking 'drugs' available at chemists are inactive and act as a placebo, providing a prop or encouragement. Dummy cigarettes fall into this category.

◆ If you decide that you really want to give up smoking, get help and support from your family, doctor, and, if possible, a nearby group. There is no secret method. All the above ways have been found helpful by some and it is a case of choosing a method that seems likely to suit you.

Although there is no easy way, some of the following may ease things for you:

◆ Try to find someone who you can stop smoking with. Your partner, parents, or children would be ideal helpers. It's a good idea for all members of the family to try to stop at once. If necessary, get sponsors or make a bet.

◆ Speak to your doctor and access one of the expanding services from the NHS designed to help individuals stop.

◆ Ask your family to be patient and to support you. Warn them that you may have mood swings and be less tolerant. Tell them when you are going to stop in advance so they can support you.

◆ About 2 weeks before you plan to stop, change your brand—the change in taste may help to reduce your enjoyment and thus stimulate you further to stop.

◆ Pick a quiet day to stop. Get rid of *all* ashtrays, cigarettes, and lighters the night before.

◆ STOP smoking. That means no cigarettes at all. Most studies suggest that stopping suddenly is better than gradually reducing your cigarette consumption.

◆ Try to find something to do at the danger times when you normally had a cigarette—after meals, while watching television, etc. As well as these new activities, try to find something to do with your hands.

◆ If you do crave a cigarette, go and find something else to do. Just sitting worrying about it won't work. Try to find your own distraction. After some weeks the craving will gradually decrease, as will the irritability and lack of concentration that often accompany stopping smoking.

◆ Learn to relax. Some groups can give help with relaxation exercises, and audio media are available. Hypnosis may be helpful.

◆ Don't let anyone persuade you that 'one won't hurt'. Part of you will be happy to have a cigarette and the first time you give in could be the end of the road. Friends can often be your worst enemy; you will have to put up with their jokes and temptations. Avoid places, such as pubs, where you are likely to meet such 'friends'.

- Many people worry about putting on weight when they stop smoking. This could happen because:
  - Nicotine suppresses your appetite and makes your body burn calories faster. Smoking affects your taste and smell, so food may be much tastier when you quit.
- Some people replace cigarettes with snacks and sweets when they give up. Try to eat a balanced diet and do regular, moderate, physical exercise.
- Arrange to reward yourself in ways that don't involve food or drink when you reach goals. For instance, after a month without cigarettes you can afford a reward from the money you have saved!
- Imagine the possible consequences of starting smoking again—think of it as like playing Russian roulette.
- Keep working at it. Stopping smoking is not just a passive process.

Keep telling yourself why you are stopping. Find things to do when you need a cigarette. Take exercise. Save the money you would have spent so that you can see it grow. Work together with your family and, if possible, your doctor or a group. Don't relax after a few weeks. The only really important factor in stopping is your motivation and reasons; any other help is secondary. To be successful you must need to stop smoking more than you need the next cigarette.

Staying stopped

Giving up smoking is hard work and it may take some people several attempts to quit for good.

Remember that nicotine is very addictive and watch out for situations where you might be tempted to have 'just one cigarette'.

Helpful information and resources

These organizations may be able to help or put you in touch with those who can.

National NHS support

Free NHS Smoking Helpline: 0800 022 4 332

Website: http://smokefree.nhs.uk/

Resources include:

- Support materials.
- Downloads of inspirational videos and stop smoking guides.
- Calculators of the costs of smoking.
- Addiction tests.
- Effects on the body.
- A promisary note for your friends and family.

Action on Smoking and Health (ASH)

First Floor, 144–145 Shoreditch High Street, London E1 6JE

Tel.: 0207 739 5902

Fax: 0207 729 4732

E-mail: enquiries@ash.org.uk

Website: http://www.ash.org.uk

QUIT

211 Old Street, London EC1V 9NR

Tel.: 020 7251 1551

Fax: 020 7251 1661

E-mail: info@quit.org.uk

Website: http://www.quit.org.uk

Quitline: 0800 00 22 00

Contact general cancer organizations (see Appendix) who may be able to give you information and find groups in your area. Talk to your GP, who will know what is available locally.

Why do people start smoking?

If everyone knows or has at least heard that smoking is such a bad thing, why do so many young people take up smoking? Most smokers start during adolescence, most frequently due to peer pressure. In spite of bans on tobacco advertising, smoking can still be perceived as 'cool'. Other reasons include trying out of curiosity, out of a sense of independence and most importantly rebelliousness. Teenagers are more likely to start if their parents or friends smoke and they see the gains as sufficient to overcome the unpleasant side-effects of starting to smoke—indeed conquering them is an apparent sign of being 'grown up'.

Although less than 1% of 11- and 12-year-old children smoke, by the age of 15 years, 1 in 5 (20%) children are regular smokers in England, despite the fact that it is illegal to sell any tobacco product to under-18s.

Childhood smoking

In 2006, 9% of children aged 11–15 years smoked at least one cigarette each week: 10% of girls and 7% of boys. A disturbing recent trend has been an increase in smoking among women and young girls; men are smoking less. Since 1986, girls have had consistently higher rates of smoking than boys: in 2006, 24% of 15-year-old girls were regular smokers compared to 16% of boys. Tobacco manufacturers, realizing this, are now producing brands aimed primarily at women. One subtle influence of current advertising programmes is to accentuate the slimness of models and, by inference, the appetite suppression of smoking.

Once established, the habit is maintained by the physical and social pleasures of smoking and the difficulty in stopping. This group of young smokers will continue to be a social influence on their friends to take up the habit and to join them in being 'grown up'. Although they may have heard of the risks of smoking they think 'it couldn't happen to me'—remember that lung cancer is a disease of middle and late life, and is far removed from adolescence.

However, campaigns to reduce smoking may be starting to work and the proportion of the population that smokes has fallen from 50% in 1960 to about 22% in 2007, and continues to fall. Despite this, attempts to dissuade teenagers from smoking often fail, and new ways of approaching the problem are being looked at. We need to persuade young people that not only may it be damaging to their future health but that it is not a 'smart' thing to do. Our children will only stop the rush to become smokers when the glamour and the fantasy that it is adult to smoke have been completely destroyed.

International tobacco control

The effects of tobacco on health and changing patterns of tobacco consumption around the world as tobacco companies target the developing world has led to a global approach to tobacco control. In May 2003, the World Health Organization (WHO) adopted the world's first public health treaty, the Framework Convention on Tobacco Control (FCTC) to provide countries with the basic tools to enact comprehensive tobacco control legislation. The key provisions include price and tax measures to reduce the demand for tobacco, and non-price measures to reduce the demand for tobacco, namely:

◆ Protection from exposure to tobacco smoke.

◆ Regulation of the contents of tobacco products.

◆ Regulation of tobacco product disclosures.

◆ Packaging and labelling of tobacco products.

◆ Education, communication, training, and public awareness.

◆ Tobacco advertising, promotion, and sponsorship.

◆ Demand reduction measures concerning tobacco dependence and cessation.

The core supply reduction provisions in the WHO FCTC are contained in articles 15–17:

◆ Illicit trade in tobacco products.

◆ Sales to and by young people.

◆ Provision of support for economically viable alternative activities.

By 31 January 2007, 143 countries had ratified the treaty which, if effectively implemented, offers the possibility of stemming the tobacco pandemic in the developing world.

Many industrialized countries now have legislation to reduce the impact of tobacco on other people through the effects of passive smoking, in other words inhaling other people's tobacco fumes. In addition there are major efforts to try to reduce adolescent children becoming addicted to tobacco. The peak age of starting smoking is in the teen years despite a ban on sales to children. Clearly, stopping the young from starting smoking is essential.

Recent measures in the UK have included:

◆ The introduction of 'smoke-free' legislation in the UK was complete by 1 July 2007. This has stopped smoking in public places, both in and out of doors. Similar policies are either in place or being instituted in much of Europe.

◆ Price increases through taxation have proved to be an effective measure for reducing smoking.

◆ Tobacco advertising, promotion, and sponsorship is banned in the UK.

◆ Health warnings have to cover 30% of the front and 40% of the back of tobacco packaging.

◆ Terms such as 'low tar' and 'light' are prohibited.

◆ Maximum yields are set on the amounts of tar (10 mg), carbon monoxide (10 mg), and nicotine (1 mg) in cigarettes.

◆ The NHS Stop Smoking Service was established in 1999.

◆ The legal age to buy cigarettes has risen from 16 to 18 years in England and Wales.

Does tobacco control work? The public perception of smokers and smoking seems crucially to be changing. Smoking is now starting to be perceived by both the public and even by smokers as antisocial, i.e. as having to go outside in the cold. This is a complete turnaround in the last 20 years.

5

How lung cancer is diagnosed

➡ Key points

◆ Lung cancer can cause symptoms within the chest such as cough and breathlessness and general non-specific effects such as tiredness and ill-health.

◆ Lung cancer can cause symptoms such as pains in the bones if it spreads.

◆ A biopsy is taken to confirm that lung cancer is present and also to determine the type of lung cancer so treatment can be planned.

◆ Screening for lung cancer is not yet routine practice or of proven value.

Most cases of lung cancer are only discovered when people go to their doctor feeling unwell. However, about 1 in 20 tumours may be found incidentally on a routine chest X-ray taken for another reason.

Symptoms of the common types of lung cancer

Lung cancer in its earliest phase causes either no ill effects at all, or vague generalized symptoms such as tiredness and feeling generally unwell that are difficult to pinpoint. As the tumour grows it starts to cause symptoms, usually due to its invasion into the tissue of the lung and airways. To begin with these symptoms are often intermittent and are brought on or worsened by physical exertion. They gradually become more continuous and new problems start to appear. Often, these symptoms seem to be caused by a 'chest infection' that does not respond to the usual antibiotics and it is only when a chest X-ray is taken that the cancer is found.

The most important and common symptoms of lung cancer are shown in Figure 5.1. Many could be caused by any chest disease or infection but a few, such as coughing up blood (known as haemoptysis), are reason for immediate investigation. About two in every five patients have a cough as their first

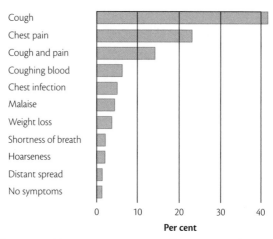

Figure 5.1 Frequency of the common symptoms of lung cancer at the time of diagnosis.

symptom and virtually all have a cough at some stage in the development of the cancer. The cough is usually persistent or recurs intermittently, often beginning with an ordinary cold or chest infection but continuing long after the signs of the cold are gone. Anyone who has a persistent cough for some weeks should, therefore, see a doctor. It is no good just calling it a 'smoker's cough'—a new and persistent cough, or a subtle change in an existing cough, needs to be explained.

Cough

Coughing is caused by stimulation of sensory nerves in the lining of the airways, anywhere from the vocal cords in the voice box (larynx) down to the small airways (bronchi) in the lungs (Figure 5.2). It is an involuntary act (reflex), although it can be started voluntarily. Coughing greatly raises the pressure in the chest and the sudden expiration of air is designed to clear away mucous secretions from the lining (mucosa) of the airways. Cancer invading the mucosa of the airways irritates the nerves and starts the cough, which fails to remove the source of irritation—the cancer—and the cough becomes persistent. Any bleeding is very irritant to the lining of the bronchi and will cause blood to be coughed up.

Paroxysms or bouts of coughing may occur if the irritation is bad and cannot be cleared. These paroxysms can be so severe as to crack a rib (a cough fracture) or damage small blood vessels in the lungs. The cough caused by lung cancer is not characteristic but it is often most noticeable at night or first thing in the morning. Later it becomes intermittent throughout the day and paroxysmal. Exertion or deep breathing will often start a coughing fit. Early in the disease

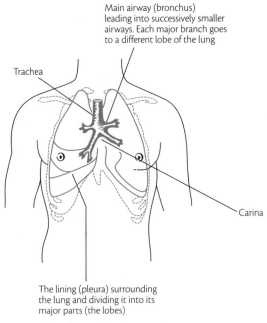

Main airway (bronchus)
leading into successively smaller
airways. Each major branch goes
to a different lobe of the lung

Trachea

Carina

The lining (pleura) surrounding
the lung and dividing it into its
major parts (the lobes)

Figure 5.2 Anatomy of the chest, major airways, and lungs.

the cough is dry but a white mucoid sputum may later be coughed up. If an infection develops this may become a purulent green or yellow and there may be blood in the sputum (haemoptysis) at any stage.

Haemoptysis usually results in some blood-streaking of sputum but if (as occasionally happens) a small vein is invaded, fresh blood may be coughed up: it is very rare for there to be severe bleeding. Haemoptysis is a very important symptom that should never be ignored and up to one in every four people over the age of 40 years who coughs up blood turns out to have lung cancer.

Chest discomfort and pain

This is the second most common initial symptom, occurring in about one in five cases. Often it is difficult to determine the nature of the pain or discomfort, which can be very variable. The most common description is of fullness and pressure, which is worse in certain positions and on deep breathing or coughing. There may occasionally be a sharp localized pain in the chest on breathing or coughing (pleuritic pain); this is due to inflammation of the lining over the lung (the pleura).

Tumours high in the upper part of the lungs may affect the large nerve roots (brachial plexus) at the base of the neck and can cause progressive pain in the upper chest, shoulder, and upper arm.

Chest infection and obstruction

Growth of tumour in the larger airways of the lung may gradually result in increasing obstruction of the airway itself. This prevents the normal mucous of the lung being coughed up and these trapped secretions often become the site for an infection. This causes malaise, chills, fevers, night sweats, and loss of appetite and weight. Infections may respond poorly to conventional antibiotics and, if complete obstruction of the airway ensues, severe shortness of breath, cough, and fevers may develop. The symptoms and their severity depend on how much of the lung is affected.

If the obstruction is incomplete it may cause a wheeze as the air tries to get past the blockage. This is worse on deep breathing, especially after exercise.

Shortness of breath

Shortness of breath is rarely the first symptom of lung cancer, although it is common during the course of the disease. There are various causes which include:

- asthma-like episodes caused by spasm of the airways;
- collapse of the lung caused by obstruction of a major airway (see above);
- infection in the lung;
- fluid between the lung and chest wall (pleural effusion; page 95);
- pressure on the major veins around the heart (superior vena caval obstruction; page 94), which also causes swelling of the neck veins and face and is made worse by bending forwards;
- collection of fluid in the sac around the heart (pericardial effusion), which restricts the heart's ability to work normally.

Hoarseness

One of the nerves going to the voice box (larynx) loops down to the root of the left lung in the centre of the chest. A tumour growing in this part of the chest may damage the nerve so that the vocal chords on that side no longer work. This causes a weak, hoarse voice and a typical brassy cough.

Distant spread and metabolic effects

The tumour may cause general effects—fever, chills, and malaise—because of infection. Less well understood are general symptoms and physical changes that are not directly related to spread of this cancer; these are often called paraneoplastic syndromes. It is presumed that they are caused by proteins or similar substances produced by the tumour or metabolic changes in the body. They include:

◆ *Skin changes.* These can be very variable but the two most common are a dark rash under the arms or around the neck and upper chest (called acanthosis nigricans) and a skin rash associated with progressive muscle weakness and discomfort (called dermatomyositis).

◆ *Bone changes.* The most common of these is clubbing—thickening of the finger tips, with typical nail changes. More generalized bone changes (pulmonary hypertrophic osteoarthropathy) can cause painful swelling in the joints of bones of the arms and legs. These symptoms sometimes appear several months before the diagnosis of lung cancer is made.

◆ *Effects on the nervous system.* All sorts of effects on the nervous system can be seen in patients with lung cancer and these may precede detection of the lung cancer by quite long periods. The most common of these effects is weakness or unsteadiness on walking or getting up from a sitting position (page 102).

◆ *Production of excessive amount of hormones.* Some lung tumours produce normal hormones in excessive amounts and may cause symptoms because of this (page 97).

Remember that all of these effects are rather rare and the chances of anyone with a rash or bone problem turning out to have lung cancer is exceedingly small.

Secondary or metastatic spread

Tumours of the lung can also spread outside the chest in the lymphatic system or in the blood (page 4). Symptoms of spread are relatively uncommon as the first evidence of the disease but may develop during the course of the illness. The common sites of spread are:

◆ Lymph glands in the neck, which become involved in up to half of cases. They can be felt as firm lumps at the root of the neck.

◆ Bones, especially the spine, ribs, skull, and limb bones, may become involved in up to 40% of cases.

◆ Spread to the liver is uncommon at first but may develop in up to half of patients.

◆ Spread to the brain may occur late in the course of the disease (page 100).

Other parts of the lungs can be affected in up to one third of patients.

Tests used to diagnose lung cancer

If, after a doctor has heard all about the patient's symptoms and has completed an examination, there is any suspicion of lung cancer, a chest X-ray must be taken immediately. A chest X-ray gives a two-dimensional picture (a photographic negative) of the chest and shows up the different organs by their varying densities. Hence, the dense, blood-filled heart is seen as a white area, which contrasts with the dark, air-filled lungs. A tumour, or an area of infection, increases the density of the bit of lung affected and will show up as a denser white area or shadow. By the time lung cancer is suspected the patient's chest X-ray is nearly always abnormal. However, it is impossible for the doctor to know exactly what the abnormal shadow is—it could be infection or many other things—and, even if it is a tumour, an X-ray cannot tell what type it is and the doctor cannot be sure that it started in the lung.

It is, therefore, essential that a bit of the abnormal area or tumour is obtained for examination under a microscope. The test used to do this will depend on exactly where the tumour is.

Microscopic examination

Microscopic examination (cytology) of sputum that has been coughed up may be used to diagnose lung cancer. Cancer cells may be seen in the sputum and, together with a typical chest X-ray, can be used to make the diagnosis of lung cancer. However, doctors will always prefer to have the greater accuracy and confidence gained by examining a piece of the tumour itself (a biopsy).

Biopsy of a lymph node

If, on examination, an abnormal lymph gland is found (usually at the root of the neck), it is worth taking a sample of this for examination as it gives the best chance of making a firm diagnosis. This is usually done with a needle and syringe rather like taking a blood sample.

Pleural biopsy

If there is fluid between the lung and chest wall (pleural effusion), a piece of the pleural lining of the chest may be removed for examination under a microscope. When the fluid is being removed (page 95) a special needle is used to cut away a small piece of the pleura. Although this is done after an injection of local anaesthetic, it can be uncomfortable and a sedative may be required to help reduce any discomfort. Increasingly these biopsies are targeted to abnormal areas during a computed tomography (CT) scan.

Bronchoscopy

Approximately 70% of all lung cancers affect the proximal main airways and will be accessible by a bronchoscopy. This means using a tube to look down into the main airways of the lungs (Figure 5.2, page 37). In the past a metal tube (a rigid bronchoscope) was used requiring a general anaesthetic, but now a thin flexible bronchoscope is usually passed after some short-acting sedative has been given. This flexible bronchoscope, using either video or nowadays optical fibres, allows the doctor to look directly into the airways.

When the bronchoscope is in the major airways it is possible to take a small piece of tissue for examination (a biopsy). In addition a brush or sponge can be rubbed against the walls of the airways to collect cells that can be examined microscopically. Cells may also be washed out in a small amount of fluid. Using these methods, most cancers can be diagnosed with great accuracy.

Bronchoscopy is usually done in hospital as a day case procedure. Before a flexible bronchoscope is used, an injection of a short-acting sedative is given into a vein and an anaesthetic spray is used on the back of the throat. The patient is half awake when this test is done, the thin bronchoscope being passed through a nostril into the back of the throat and then down into the lungs. A few hours after the test the patient may go home, but should not drive because of the sedative or anaesthetic injection they have recently received. Following the test, some patients have a sore throat and a few cough up a little blood.

Aspiration of lung tissue

In the case of a suspicious lump in the periphery of the lungs, which is beyond the reach of a bronchoscope, a thin needle may be passed through the skin into the lung itself. Patients are asked to stop breathing for a short time while this is done and a tiny piece of lung tissue is aspirated—sucked out of the lung. The test is done under X-ray control, increasingly on the CT scanner so that the needle can be guided to the suspicious area, and experienced doctors have a high rate of success in getting a small piece of lung tissue to make the diagnosis. Leakage of air into the space between the lung and chest wall (pneumothorax; page 95) occurs in about 1 in 5 cases but in most it is not serious. Removal of this air is either not necessary if very small or can often be removed using a needle and syringe. Very rarely patients have to be admitted to hospital to have the air removed with a drainage tube (page 61). Occasionally patients cough up some blood after the test has been done.

Exploratory operation

In those few patients (usually with a small single suspicious area in the periphery of the lung called a nodule), where it is not possible to make a diagnosis using the above tests, an exploratory operation (thoracotomy) can be done to examine the lung. As more patients have whole body CT scans for other medical reasons this is becoming a more frequent practice. As this group of patients, if it is lung cancer, form the group who are potentially most easily cured by an operation to remove the tumour, it is important not to just wait and see what happens on repeated X-rays. However, not all nodules are cancerous and opening the chest is a major operation. The appearances on the CT scan, and now in some instances positron emission tomography (PET) scans, including size and shape of the nodule can be used to determine the risk of that nodule being cancer and tell doctors whether it should be removed immediately or can be followed with repeat scans at planned intervals usually of a few months.

If it remains possible that the shadow could be cancer and all the other tests are unhelpful, an operation to remove the lump should be done.

Exploratory operation for microscopic examination of lymph glands

Where there are enlarged, suspicious glands in the centre of the chest, an exploratory minor operation (mediastinoscopy or mediastinotomy; page 51) may be undertaken to remove a gland for microscopic examination.

Screening for lung cancer

Because lung cancer is most curable when it is caught in its earliest stages, attempts have been made to screen healthy people to see if it is possible to detect lung cancers before they cause symptoms. The idea is that the patients found on screening to have an early cancer will stand a better chance of cure.

There are, unfortunately, no reliable blood tests that can be used to detect lung cancer at an early stage. Other screening tests have consisted of getting people to cough up sputum samples for cytology (page 40) and then having a chest X-ray. These studies tended to find that screening detects malignant tumours at an earlier stage but there was no evidence that those people in the screening group stood a better chance of being cured.

The widespread introduction of CT scanners has led to trials in high risk groups such as lifelong smokers or those with chronic bronchitis. CT scans are much more sensitive than chest X-rays for identifying lung cancers and can also identify a significantly higher proportion of small (early stage, operable) lung cancers than ordinary X-rays. However, the effectiveness of CT scans in reducing deaths from lung cancer is not yet known, because of the absence of randomization and the lack of an unscreened control group for which mortality was an outcome in the studies performed to date. Researchers in the USA are trying to find out whether screening with spiral CT scanning would help them diagnose lung cancer earlier and improve the cure rate. This is a large trial, involving 50,000 people, and will take some years to determine whether this approach reduces the risk of death from lung cancer. All health screening has obvious potential benefits in reducing death rates from cancer. However, there is also risk of harm in the discomfort both physically and mentally when the test shows an abnormality that turns out not to be cancer, i.e. a false-positive screening test. Further tests sometimes including surgery may be necessary. The false-positive rates with CT scans range from 5% to 40%, but fortunately most can be resolved with further CT scans.

At present, large-scale screening of the general population for lung cancer is not generally recommended.

6

Tests used to stage lung cancer

> ## ⮕ Key points
>
> ◆ The extent of the disease is known as the 'stage', and this helps to plan treatment and indicate likely prognosis.
>
> ◆ The extent of investigation varies according to general health and possible treatments but is likely to include a computed tomography (CT) scan.
>
> ◆ Measures of patients' fitness help to select treatments that can be tolerated.
>
> ◆ Uniform staging systems help healthcare professionals communicate about patients and also present their results.

'Staging' is a term used to describe the process of assessing the extent of spread and growth of a malignant tumour. It is done to help select the best treatment and to gain an idea of the patient's outlook or prognosis from the disease. The degree of spread of most cancers is described by a staging system, which defines how big a tumour has grown, and how far it has spread. The worldwide use of uniform staging systems also allows doctors to discuss and compare results of treatments in different groups of patients. Lung cancer is no exception.

As the approach to treatment is different for small cell and non-small cell lung cancer, there are separate staging systems for each.

Small cell cancer

Since surgery is rarely used in the treatment of this cancer, a very simple system of staging is used:

◆ *Limited stage*. Disease confined to one side of the chest. Disease may be very extensive within that side of the chest compared with the TNM system; page 44) and to the draining lymph nodes on that side (including those at the root of the neck).

◆ *Extensive stage*. Any disease that has spread beyond this (including distant lymph nodes, bone, liver, bone marrow, brain, etc.).

Chemotherapy is the mainstay of treatment for this tumour and the major distinction between limited and extensive disease is more important in understanding the patient's prognosis and need for radiotherapy. For many the practical definition of limited disease is therefore one where the disease is contained within a volume that can be treated by radiotherapy (page 79).

Non-small cell cancer

Surgery is the most important treatment in non-small cell lung cancer and traditionally it is considered the only possible truly curative measure. For this reason the staging system used is much more complicated because it has to give a detailed estimate of the size and distribution of the tumour (see box below). This is known as a TNM system: T stands for tumour size, N for lymph nodes, and M for metastases (the distant spread of tumour). The importance of such a staging system is in selecting those patients who will benefit from an operation to remove part or all of the lung and the cancer within it. Clearly only those with a small tumour and with little or no spread to lymph nodes and no spread to other parts of the body will stand a chance of cure with an operation.

This staging system was last updated in 2004 and reflects information and outcome from many thousands of patients.

Simplified staging system for non-small cell lung cancer (TNM 6)

Primary tumour (T)

T1   Tumour <3 cm in diameter, surrounded by normal lung, and not invading the lung more centrally than before the airway leading to that segment of the lung (the lobular bronchus).

T2   Tumour >3 cm and <7 cm in diameter, or any size if invading the pleura or associated with some lung collapse or infection. Any such tumour must be >2 cm away from the main division of the major airway (carina; Figure 5.2).

T3   Tumours >7 cm in diameter or of any size invading the chest wall, the diaphragm (muscular wall between chest and abdomen), the area around the heart and major blood vessels, or tumour within 2 cm of the carina, or collapse of an entire lung, or a pleural effusion.

Draining lymph nodes (N)

N0   No spread to the draining lymph nodes.

N1   Spread to the first group of draining lymph nodes at the lung hilum.

N2   Spread into the lymph nodes in the centre of the chest: the mediastinum.

Distant metastases (M)

M0   No known metastases.

M1   Distant metastases found including pleural or pericardial effusion.

The extent of disease estimated by TNM is used to group patients into four stages, those with the least disease being designated stage 1 and those with the most disease stage 4.

Table 6.1 Lung cancer stage groupings and 5-year survival

Stage	TNM	5-year survival
IA	T1N0M0	75%
IB	T2N0M0	55%
IIA	T1N1M0	40%
IIB	T2N1M0 or T3N0M0	40%
IIIA	T1-3N2M0 or T3N1M0	10–35%
IIIB	Any T4 or any N3M0	5%
IV	Any M1	<5%

One of the most striking features of lung cancer compared to many other cancers is the relatively low cure rates even when the disease is discovered in the early stages. For example, stage 1 colon cancer has a 5-year survival in excess of 90%.

In 2009 it is likely that this staging system will change slightly to reflect modern treatment outcomes.

Proposed changes to TNM staging (version 7)

Primary tumour (T)

♦ T1 lesions are divided based upon size into T1a (≤2 cm) and T1b (>2 cm but <3 cm).

♦ T2 lesions are divided into T2a (≤5 cm) and T2b (>5 cm but ≤7 cm).

♦ T2 tumours >7 cm are reclassified as T3.

♦ T4 tumours with satellite nodules in the same lobe as the primary tumour are reclassified as T3.

- Additional nodules in a different lobe of same lung are reclassified as T4 rather than M1.

- Malignant pleural or pericardial effusions or pleural nodules are now classified as metastasis (M1a) rather than T4.

Regional nodes (N)

- No changes.

Metastasis (M)

- Subdivided into M1a (malignant pleural or pericardial effusion, pleural nodules, nodules in contralateral lung) and M1b (distant metastasis).

Stage grouping

- T2aN1M0 lesions are classified as IIA, rather than IIB.

- T2bN0M0 lesions are classified as IIA, rather than IB.

- T3 (>7 cm), N0M0 lesions are classified as IIB, rather than IB.

- T3 (>7 cm), N1M0 lesions are classified as IIIA, rather than IIB.

- T3N0M0 (nodules in same lobe) lesions are classified as IIB, rather than IIIB.

- T3N1M0 or T3N2M0 (nodules in same lobe) are classified as IIIA, rather than IIIB.

- T4M0 (ipsilateral lung nodules) lesions are classified as IIIA (if N0 or N1) and IIIB (if N2 or N3), rather than stage IV.

- T4M0 (direct extension) lesions are classified as IIIA (if N0 or N1), rather than IIIB.

- Malignant pleural effusions (M1a) are classified as IV, rather than IIIB.

Staging tests

The aims of staging in non-small cell lung cancer are to define the extent of the primary tumour in the lung and to decide if it has spread locally to lymph nodes in the chest or to distant parts of the body. Although we place great confidence in modern scans and techniques, the reality is that all tests in medicine can give what turns out to be either a correct or an incorrect result. The chance of giving a correct result is called the sensitivity of the test. The specificity of a test is the likelihood of recognising the abnormality correctly as cancerous, for example. Doing more than one test increases both the sensitivity and specificity of investigations. Thus if the doctors are worried about the test results, further investigations are likely to be suggested.

Staging tests prior to treatment in non-small cell lung cancer (appropriate patients will be selected to have some of these tests)

All patients

- Physical examination.
- Chest X-ray.
- Blood tests.
- Bronchoscopy or biopsy through the skin on a CT scanner.
- Biopsy of a gland or obvious tumour mass if present.

Patients in whom an operation is considered possible

- CT scan of chest and upper abdomen including the liver.
- PET scan.
- Mediastinoscopy or mediastinotomy in highly selected patients.
- Needle biopsy of the tumour in selected patients.
- Lung function tests.
- Heart tests such as exercise test or echocardiogram (an ultrasound examination of the heart).

Staging tests prior to treatment in small cell lung cancer

- Chest X-ray.
- Blood tests.
- Bronchoscopy.
- CT scan of chest and upper abdomen.

Chest X-ray

The size and position of the primary tumour (T) can be initially gauged from chest X-rays (Figure 6.1) and by looking directly into the airways to the lungs (bronchoscopy; see below). The chest X-ray will show the size and location of the tumour and whether there is associated lung collapse or infection. Sometimes it can show spread to other parts of the lung or bone.

Bronchoscopy

This defines how near the tumour is to the division of the main airway or bronchus. If too close (typically ≤2 cm) the tumour is considered inoperable.

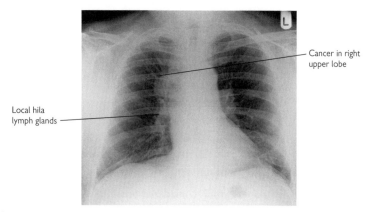

Cancer in right upper lobe

Local hila lymph glands

Figure 6.1 Chest X-ray appearances of lung cancer.

Computed tomography (CT) scan

This is an X-ray technique that uses information built up in three dimensions by a computer rather than an ordinary X-ray film. CT scanning is now the most common staging test used for lung cancer. Most modern machines take a series of pictures through the whole chest by a spiral technique that takes only a few seconds. The computer-produced picture is much better than ordinary X-rays in defining small structures. Additional information on the situation and size of the primary cancer in the lung will also be gained from a CT scan, and it can show enlarged lymph glands in the centre of the chest, as well as spread to other organs such as the liver or adrenal glands. However, if a CT scan shows that the lymph glands in the centre of the chest (mediastinum) are enlarged, they are not always later confirmed as being cancerous. In addition, up to one-quarter of patients whose glands do not appear to be enlarged also turn out to contain cancer cells, so the test is not absolute. An intravenous injection of contrast medium is usually given and this shows up in the scans in the major blood vessels. This often helps to tell the difference between a small blood vessel and a lymph gland. It also improves the sensitivity of the scan in detecting spread to other organs, particularly the liver (Figure 6.2).

Positron emission tomography (PET) scan

This type of scan was developed in the 1970s. It can show how body tissues are working, as well as what they look like. With a PET scan an injection of a very small amount of radioactive drug (tracer) is given. The amount of radiation is very small—no more than that received having a normal chest X-ray. The isotope only stays in the body for a few hours. The most common drug or isotope used is fluorine 18, also known as FDG-18. This is a radioactive version

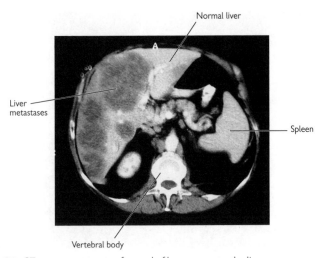

Normal liver

Liver metastases

Spleen

Vertebral body

Figure 6.2 CT scan appearances of spread of lung cancer to the liver.

of glucose. When FDG-18 is injected into your body it travels to places where glucose is used for energy. It shows up cancers because they use glucose in a different way from normal tissue. PET scans also show up changes in tissues that use glucose as their main source of energy, for example the brain. PET scans are usually done at the same time as a CT scan. If there is a lump visible on the CT scan, the PET part of the scan shows whether there are actively dividing cells taking up radioisotope (Figure 6.3). If so, these are likely to be cancerous. Abnormalities that do not take up the isotope are statistically relatively unlikely to be cancerous. PET scans can show further spread of the cancer in up to one-third of cases compared to CT scans alone, and are now considered a compulsory test if surgery is being contemplated.

Mediastinoscopy

An enlarged lymph node found in the chest on CT scan, whether or not it takes up PET isotope, is not always cancerous. Often the only way to be sure is to take a small sample from these lymph nodes. Sometimes this can be through the bronchoscope or oesophagoscope using a process known as endoluminal ultrasound. Here an ultrasound probe is attached to the end of the scope. If a swollen lymph gland is detected, a small sample can be taken through a needle guided by the ultrasound probe. More commonly, however, a minor surgical procedure known as mediastinoscopy is undertaken.

Mediastinoscopy requires a general anaesthetic. A small incision is made at the base of the neck, just above the breast bone (Figure 6.4). A special instrument—the mediastinoscope—is passed through the incision into the upper chest.

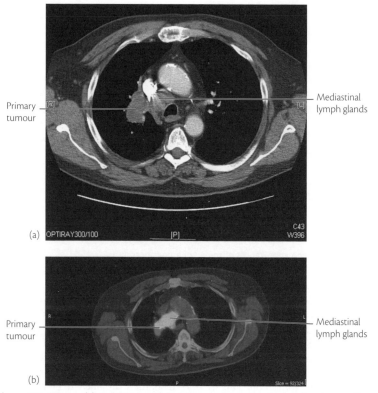

Primary tumour — Mediastinal lymph glands

(a)

Primary tumour — Mediastinal lymph glands

(b)

Figure 6.3 CT scan (a) and PET scan (b) of the same case showing locally advanced lung cancer. The chest X-ray in Figure 6.1 is the same case.

It shines a light into the chest and the chest surgeon can look through it to examine the area around the lungs and heart—the area known as the mediastinum. The surgeon can also take a sample (biopsy) of any suspicious areas. This test picks up most abnormal lymph nodes in the top area of the centre of the chest and it is important to perform mediastinoscopy because an operation to remove the cancer will not be successful if more than one or two groups of these mediastinal nodes contain cancer.

Mediastinotomy

This can be used as an alternative to mediastinoscopy if the lymph nodes are not accessible by the mediastinoscope, or if mediastinoscopy fails to give all the information needed. Under general anaesthetic a small operation is done to open the front of the chest, usually between the second and third ribs, on the side where the cancer is growing (Figure 6.5). The advantage of this method is

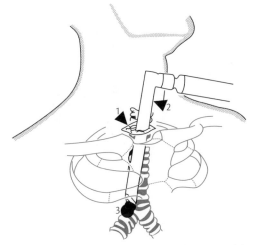

Figure 6.4 Mediastinoscopy. A cut is made at the base of the throat (1) and the instrument (2) is passed into the space in the upper chest to look at the glands (3).

that it provides a more direct approach to the mediastinal glands, which can be examined with or without a mediastinoscope. These tests may be used either to make the diagnosis of cancer if no other biopsy can be taken or to see whether the mediastinal lymph nodes are involved if an operation is being planned.

Other tests used in staging lung cancer

Blood tests

There is no blood test that can accurately and reliably diagnose lung cancer. Sometimes patients with lung cancer can become anaemic due to their illness. A simple blood test can detect this by measuring the haemoglobin level. Blood taken from a vein in the arm is also used to see how well the liver is working. However, these tests are not very specific as many factors can affect the way the liver is working. When used together with other tests described below, they can, however, add useful information. Blood tests may also be useful because a chemical derived from bone—alkaline phosphatase—may be present in increased amounts when the bones are involved with cancer. The amount of calcium in the blood is also measured, as high levels will make the patient unwell (page 98).

Barium swallow

For some patients the extent of lymph node spread in the chest can press on the gullet (oesophagus) and stop patients being able to swallow food. These lymph glands may be visible on CT scan but also during a barium swallow when some

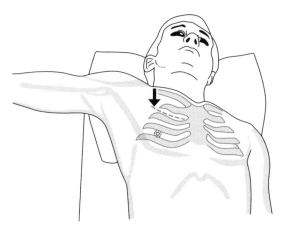

Figure 6.5 Typical site for the cut used for mediastinotomy. This may be on either side of the chest.

white dye is swallowed and then a series of X-rays taken to follow the dye pass into the stomach. This dye or contrast medium outlines the oesophagus and shows any enlarged lymph nodes or tumour that may be pressing against or invading the oesophagus.

Ultrasound scans of the liver

In this test, a source of high-frequency sound waves (well beyond what the human ear can hear) is pressed lightly over the part of the body to be examined. The beam of sound waves is bounced back off the various parts of the liver and a computer builds up a picture of the liver according to its varying consistency. Tumours show as areas where there are changes in consistency or density of the liver tissue. This test is very simple, painless, and easily repeated.

Isotope bone scan

One commonly used test to show spread of cancer to the bones is an isotope bone scan. A radioactive isotope called technetium-99m, which is absorbed by bones, is injected into a vein and a picture of the skeleton then taken with a gamma camera. The amount of radiation is small. It is similar to that from an X-ray examination. The radioactivity will disappear by itself soon after the scan is finished (nearly all of it disappears within one day, any remaining traces disappear within one week). Most cancers in bones take up more of the isotope than normal bone and they therefore appear on the picture as a bright 'hot' spot. Occasionally it may fail to take up the isotope and can be seen as a cold spot, or hole. Bone scans often detect tumour up to 18 months before anything can be seen on an X-ray and they are therefore one of the best ways to look at the bones when staging a cancer. However, they also detect the amount of bone repair that is going on, so arthritis and injuries often show up. Skilled interpretation of the images produced can usually distinguish benign problems from malignant cancers on an abnormal scan.

The brain: magnetic resonance imaging (MRI) scan or CT scan

Unfortunately some lung tumours do spread to the brain, although it is unusual for the brain to be involved when cancer is first diagnosed. Because of this, tests to look for brain metastases are not normally done unless the patient has symptoms suggesting that there may be a problem (page 100). CT or MRI scans may be used to see if the tumour is involving the brain.

CT scan performed after the administration of an intravenous injection of contrast is the usual way of looking for tumour in the brain. The test is simple and painless, although the injection of X-ray contrast dye, which may be used to outline a tumour, will cause a hot flush for a few minutes.

MRI scans

Magnetic resonance imaging has been used since the beginning of the 1980s. The MRI scan uses magnetic and radio waves, meaning that there is no exposure to X-rays or any other damaging forms of radiation. You lie inside a large, cylinder-shaped magnet. Radio waves 10,000 to 30,000 times stronger than the magnetic field of the earth are then sent through the body. This affects the body's atoms, forcing the nuclei into a different position. As they move back into place they send out radio waves of their own. The scanner picks up these signals and a computer turns them into a picture. These pictures are based on the location and strength of the incoming signals. The scans are painless and entirely harmless.

MRI scanners tend to be more intimidating for patients because you have to get into a confined space. In addition the equipment is noisy and complex which can be rather daunting. The images produced can be made from different angles—an advantage over CT imaging, which can only view from one direction.

As well as MRI scans of the brain to show up spread there, MRI can also be used to increase the sensitivity and specificity of other tests. For example, MRI scans with heavy metal contrast can help to determine whether an abnormality shown in the liver is cancerous or not.

The adrenal glands sit on top of the kidneys and are one of the commonest places that lung cancer spreads to. A benign adenoma that causes no ill-effects is a common finding within the general population. The phase of MRI scans can help determine whether that lump is an adenoma or cancer.

MRI scans are also used for tumours at the top of the chest known as superior sulcus or pancoast tumours. These tumours commonly invade into the chest wall or press on nerves where they exit the vertebral column or spine. The local extent of the tumour is best shown on MRI.

MRI scan is the most sensitive test for spread of cancer to bone. Bone scanning is often initially preferred because it can look at all the bones in the body, whereas MRI scans can only look at one or possibly two areas at one examination.

Performance status

One other vital piece of information is how fit any patient is, otherwise known as performance status. This has been shown to have prognostic significance, independent of the stage of the disease as described above. Perhaps this is not surprising as unfit patients, often with other major medical problems, will not be able to tolerate aggressive treatments. Doctors use scoring systems to determine performance status. The two commonly used are described in the boxes below.

WHO performance status

The Eastern Cooperative Oncology Group (ECOG) score, also called the WHO or Zubrod score, runs from 0 to 5, with 0 denoting perfect health and 5 death:

0   Asymptomatic (fully active, able to carry on all pre-disease activities without restriction).

1   Symptomatic but completely ambulatory (restricted in physically strenuous activity but ambulatory and able to carry out work of a light or sedentary nature. For example, light housework, office work).

2   Symptomatic, <50% in bed during the day (ambulatory and capable of all self-care but unable to carry out any work activities. Up and active >50% of waking hours).

3   Symptomatic, >50% in bed, but not bed-bound (capable of only limited self-care, confined to bed or chair ≥50% of waking hours).

4   Bed-bound (completely disabled; cannot carry on any self-care; totally confined to bed or chair).

5   Death.

From: Oken MM, Creech RH, Tormey DC, Horton J, Davis TE, McFadden ET, Carbone PP. Toxicity and response criteria of the Eastern Cooperative Oncology Group. Am J Clin Oncol 1982;5:649–6. © Eastern Cooperative Oncology Group, Robert Comis MD, Group Chair.

Karnofsky performance status

The Karnofsky score runs from 100 to 0, where 100 is 'perfect' health and 0 is death. It is named after Dr David A. Karnofsky, who described the scale with Dr Joseph H. Burchenal in 1949.

100%	Normal, no complaints, no signs of disease.
90%	Capable of normal activity, few symptoms or signs of disease.
80%	Normal activity with some difficulty, some symptoms or signs.
70%	Caring for self, not capable of normal activity or work.
60%	Requiring some help, can take care of most personal requirements.
50%	Requires help often, requires frequent medical care.
40%	Disabled, requires special care and help.
30%	Severely disabled, hospital admission indicated but no risk of death.
20%	Very ill, urgently requiring admission, requires supportive measures or treatment.
10%	Moribund, rapidly progressive fatal disease processes.
0%	Death.

In practice, for example, the major evidence of benefit for chemotherapy in advanced disease is in patients with WHO performance status 0 or 1. Standardized staging systems and measures of performance status allow doctors to compare results and communicate about suitable treatments for individual patients.

Part 2

Treatment

We have seen that there are different types of lung cancer. A number of treatments can be used alone or in combination. Anyone with cancer is, of course, hoping for a cure, but unfortunately this is currently possible only for a small number of patients with early or small amounts of disease. Increasingly methods of screening are being sought to try to identify those patients who can be cured.

Treatment choice is largely determined by:

◆ the type of cancer;

◆ the stage or extent of the cancer;

◆ the fitness of the patient;

◆ the wishes of the patient.

Surgery or radiotherapy will often be used to try to cure a small tumour. If more extensive tumour is discovered then cure is often not possible. Treatment is then called palliative—not only to try to prolong life but also to palliate, i.e. relieve troublesome symptoms and improve the quality of life. In this scenario, treatment decisions must be governed not only by the possible benefits of treatment but, also balanced carefully against the possible side-effects of treatment.

Patients and their families usually need time to discuss what has been found by the various staging tests with their doctor. Nowadays the doctor will be a specialist member of a team charged with responsibility for diagnosing and treating patients with lung cancer. A truthful and open discussion is best for everyone to make difficult decisions at this time. The doctor should give hope where treatment can help but be truthful and realistic according to the situation.

It is hoped that this book will answer some questions that arise, but it is very important to develop an understanding, trusting relationship with your doctors and nurses. Books like this cannot and should not replace that, but can be a useful source of support and information.

Subsequent chapters will show that we have made progress in the treatment of lung cancer, nevertheless some sections may make depressing reading. They are, however, important to help patients and their relatives make decisions about their care.

7

Treatment of non-small cell lung cancer

➔ Key points

♦ The treatment is planned according to the extent of the disease and general fitness.

♦ The major curative treatment is surgery.

♦ Radiotherapy can cure lung cancer and also help the common symptoms.

♦ Chemotherapy either adds to radiotherapy or surgery for cure or is used to prolong the quantity and quality of life.

♦ Newer targeted treatments offer the hope of improving treatment outcomes with fewer side-effects.

Surgery

Non-small cell lung cancer is a grouping of at least three types of lung cancer: squamous cell, adenocarcinoma and large cell carcinoma. They are grouped together because they largely behave in a similar fashion, treatment options are almost identical, and an operation remains the best chance of cure for all three cancers. Although operations to remove a part of the lung had been attempted earlier, the first successful operation to remove a cancerous lung was done in 1933. That patient was a 48-year-old doctor who recovered well and continued to work for many years.

Operations to remove part or all of the lung are now commonly done around the world, but still carry significant risk, largely because these major operations are done on patients who are either elderly—because this is the age group that typically develops lung cancer—or have other medical problems including heart and chest problems largely related to smoking. In practice less than 10% of patients have disease that is localized enough to be suitable for surgery and who are also fit to withstand an operation.

Selection of patients for an operation

The major issue is to select patients who are most likely to benefit from a major operation despite the risks, in other words those who genuinely may be curable. Selection by staging the disease is therefore designed as much to pick out those patients who definitely stand a chance of being cured by surgery—this is discussed in Chapter 6. The recent introduction of positron emission tomography (PET) scans has led to a 15–20% reduction in patients coming for surgery because they show disease that has spread away from the lung not previously shown on other tests. These patients are then spared a major operation which cannot be of benefit. The major findings that would suggest that an operation is not going to be useful are:

◆ Cancer that has spread outside the chest or to the other lung.

◆ Cancer invading or pressing on the major airways near the main division in the chest (the carina).

◆ Cancer invading the trachea (the main airway into the chest).

◆ Invasion of the major blood vessels or heart.

◆ Involvement of multiple lymph nodes in the centre of the chest (mediastinum) or on the other side of the chest.

◆ Involvement of lymph nodes at the root of the neck.

◆ Fluid around the lungs (pleural effusion).

◆ Loss of voice and hoarseness caused by pressure on one of the nerves supplying the vocal chords in the larynx or voice box.

Lung function tests

Not only must the disease be localized to be removed surgically, but also the lungs and the heart must be able to withstand an operation. As well as simple tests of exercise tolerance, there are sophisticated ways of measuring the lung's capacity for breathing. These tests are done by patients being asked to breathe normally, and then in other tests as much as they can. This enables the anaesthetist to decide whether or not patients can withstand an operation and in particular the loss of part or whole of a lung.

Operations for non-small cell lung cancer

The two major operations performed are either lobectomy, in other words removal of part of a lung, or pneumonectomy, which is removal of a whole lung. As diagnostic tests have become more sensitive, it is increasingly unusual for patients to be found to be inoperable at the time of surgery, although this may well still be the case in up to 10% of patients. The type of operation that is done thus depends on the size of the tumour, its position, and the general health of the patient.

Traditionally tumours <2 cm from where the main airway divides were considered inoperable. The newer operation of sleeve resection can sometimes allow an operation to proceed for such cases, and also allow for lobectomy to take place when previously pneumonectomy was the only option. In a sleeve resection the ends of the airway are rejoined and any remaining lobes can be reattached. This surgery is done to save part of the lung. Sometimes a very conservative approach is taken where just part of the lung is taken. Indeed, if a small lump is visible on a chest X-ray it may be uncertain what it is, and then an excision biopsy, otherwise known as a wedge excision of a part of lung, can take place.

The aim of surgery is to remove all known disease while conserving as much normal lung as possible. In general, it is best if the lymph glands that filter the affected area of the lung are at least partially removed. This procedure reduces the risk of the cancer recurring within the chest. Also if the lymph glands are involved by cancer cells chemotherapy is likely to be suggested after the operation.

How is surgery undertaken?

Lung operations or thoracotomy can be carried out with the patient either face-up or face-down using an excision over the front or back of the chest. It is far more common, however, to place patients on their side with the tumour uppermost. The chest is opened using an incision that usually starts just below the nipple in front and curves backwards just below the tip of the shoulder blade almost to the spine. The various layers of muscle below the skin are divided and the inside of the chest is opened either by removing part of a rib or cutting through the muscles between two ribs. Having opened the chest, the surgeon is then in a position to examine the lung and its lymph nodes. It is often at this time point that the surgeon can finally decide what operation will be undertaken.

After the operation patients are carefully monitored, but you can expect the following:

◆ A drain will be left in the chest to help remove air from around the lung. This is connected to a bottle containing water that prevents air getting back into the space around the lung.

◆ Most patients need some oxygen, sometimes initially by ventilator.

◆ Physiotherapy will be started to clear secretions from the lung. This can be uncomfortable at first, even though painkillers are given. Patients need encouragement and advice on how to reduce the pain.

◆ Patients will be asked to move their legs around in bed and will get out of bed to try to reduce the risks of clots developing in the veins of the legs. A course of blood-thinning injections using a form of heparin will be given under the skin, and stockings will be fitted to the legs to further reduce the risk of blood clots.

Frequent checks of pulse, blood pressure, and breathing will be made and small samples of blood taken to check for haemoglobin and oxygen levels.

When the lung has fully re-expanded the chest tubes will be removed, and then finally after about a week the stitches. Inevitably because the chest has been opened there will be pain and discomfort and strong painkillers may be needed for some weeks after the operation.

Getting over the operation

Following the operation patients gradually increase their exercise. The pain in the chest wall from the division of a rib or muscles can persist and require painkillers for up to 18 months after the operation. Following the surgery the multidisciplinary team will meet and examine the pathology of the removed lung specimen and there will be a discussion with you to decide whether further treatment is required.

The team will discuss the pathology:

- What the tumour looks like under the microscope (the grade and type of cancer).
- Was the tumour removed completely?
- Were the lymph glands involved with cancer, if so which and how many?
- The stage of the cancer can then be conclusively known.

Complications of surgery

In spite of increasing care a small number of people will die after an operation, but many will have side-effects. This can include:

- Excessive bleeding during the operation—rarely difficult to control if patients are selected carefully.
- Changes in heart rhythm or heart attacks—again these can usually be controlled with drugs.
- Persistent leakage of air into the chest cavity requiring prolonged drainage—very occasionally another operation is needed to seal an air link from the main airway where it was tied off.
- Collapse of a part of the lung or infection.
- Infection in the chest between the lung and chest wall and empyema (an abscess) that requires drainage by a tube.
- Formation of clots in the veins of the legs, possibly breaking off and travelling to the chest; these requiring blood-thinning drugs.
- All operations have a risk of patients dying, otherwise known as the mortality rate. This is a very major operation. Current UK mortality rates for lobectomy are 7% and for pneumonectomy 10%.

Most patients, however, will have few problems and can leave hospital within 2 weeks.

Results of surgery

The results of surgery are determined by the stage, i.e. the extent of the disease. Table 7.1 shows survival rates after surgery for non-small cell lung cancer. In general if the tumour is going to recur it does so within the first 2 years following the operation and thus the chances of a cure increase the longer a patient survives without the cancer returning or relapsing. Relapses after 4 or 5 years are uncommon and the patient can be considered cured. There is, however, a continuing major risk of developing further tobacco-related cancers either within the chest or within the head and neck region, which can occur in up to 25% of patients. The importance of not smoking cannot be overstated to reduce this risk.

Adjuvant or additional treatments

Increasingly patients who undergo an operation for cancer will also be treated with a non-surgical treatment, commonly radiotherapy or chemotherapy. Chemotherapy can be given before (neo-adjuvant) or after surgery (adjuvant or additional).

Chemotherapy given after surgery has been shown to improve the chance of cure as measured by being alive at 5 years for lung cancer patients who undergo surgery and have lymph nodes involved by the cancer by 5%. Not all patients are well enough to have treatment after surgery. Treatment may also be given before surgery. The possible advantages are that by shrinking the tumour less lung may need to be removed at the time of surgery, and if there are microscopic or tiny deposits of the tumour elsewhere then they can be treated early. There is no agreement as to whether it is best to have chemotherapy before or after surgery.

Radiotherapy with or without chemotherapy may be recommended if not all the cancer has been removed at the time of surgery. The surgeon may have realized that he has not removed all the tumour, or more commonly it is only

Table 7.1 Survival by stage after surgery for lung cancer

Stage at operation	TNM	5-year survival
IA	T1N0M0	75%
IB	T2N0M0	55%
IIA	T1N1M0	40%
IIB	T2N1M0 or T3N0M0	40%
IIIA	T1-3N2M0 or T3N1M0	10–35%

discovered when the tumour specimen is examined under the microscope by the pathologist.

In the future the hope is that some of the newer targeted treatments will further reduce the risk of relapse of this disease but this is not currently proven.

Non-surgical treatments

For the majority of patients (90%) an operation cannot be performed, and for these patients alternative treatment such as radiotherapy or chemotherapy may be advised. For many of these patients the objective of treatment is to prolong the length of life, but also by relieving the symptoms of lung cancer to improve the quality of life. Such treatment is termed 'palliative'.

There is clearly a difference in the amount of treatment and the severity or toxicity of treatment that is acceptable with the aim of the treatment. When the aim is palliative and mainly to relieve symptoms, prolonged very toxic treatment is unlikely to be acceptable to patients or achieve its goal. By contrast, when the aim is cure, both patients and doctors will accept much more aggressive therapies.

Radiotherapy

Radiotherapy refers to the use of X-rays or radiation to treat cancer. High doses of radiation can damage cells and kill them. Radiation does this by producing damage within our genetic structure called DNA, causing various types of damage. A break in both strands of the DNA is thought to be the most important damage caused by ionizing radiation that results in cell death. If sufficient damage is done the cell is unable to repair itself adequately and then the cell may die, lose its ability to divide, or die when it next attempts to divide. It seems that the crucial difference between cancer cells and normal cells is that cancer cells have less ability to repair the DNA damage caused by radiotherapy than normal cells. However, the difference in this response varies between different tissues of the body and can be somewhat limited. Thus the total dose of radiation that can be given is limited by the amount of damage that the normal tissues adjacent to the tumour can tolerate.

External beam radiotherapy refers to treatment with a beam of ionizing radiation which originates outside the patient. This forms the bulk of treatment given for patients with lung cancer and most are given by a machine called a linear accelerator (Figure 7.1). This is a machine that works by firing high energy radio waves at a target. This collision generates a beam of ionizing radiation, called photons, which can then be focused into a beam to treat patients accurately. These machines do not contain radioactive sources. They are costly to buy and maintain and require specialist staff to oversee their clinical use. This is why radiotherapy departments are based in large cities and usually serve populations in excess of three-quarters of a million.

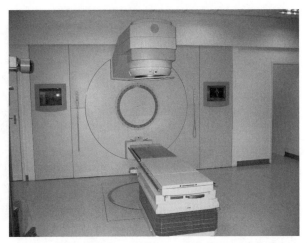

Figure 7.1 Modern megavoltage linear accelerator: radiotherapy treatment machine.

How is radiotherapy given?

Before treatment starts, the radiotherapy has to be planned. For straightforward treatments a simple X-ray will be taken on a machine called a simulator which 'simulates' the treatment position. Marks are then drawn on the chest to show the area to be treated. For more complicated treatments, a CT scan may be taken and permanent marks (tattoos) put on the skin so that the treatment can be repeated accurately each day. Following the CT scan the radiotherapist will mark the area to be treated on the CT scan, then a plan will be produced which shapes the radiation beam to the tumour in three dimensions (Figure 7.2). The objective is to treat the tumour adequately while sparing normal tissues as much as possible. Before the treatment starts there will likely be a further visit to the radiotherapy department for a process called verification which ensures the accuracy of the treatment set-up.

Treatment that is purely to relieve symptoms is commonly given in one or two treatments over a period of a week. For treatments aimed at slowing the disease or possibly curing it, treatment is given every day, Monday to Friday, over 4 to 6½ weeks. Each treatment is called a 'fraction'. A large UK trial showed that it is better to give radiotherapy over a shorter overall time (accelerated) and in more than one fraction a day (hyperfractionated). This treatment is given over 12 days, three times a day, at 8 a.m., 2 p.m., and 8 p.m. and is called CHART (Continuous Hyperfractionated Accelerated Radiation Therapy). It is only available in selected radiotherapy centres. Daily radiotherapy together with chemotherapy administered weekly or 3-weekly seems to increase the effectiveness of the radiotherapy.

Beam 1

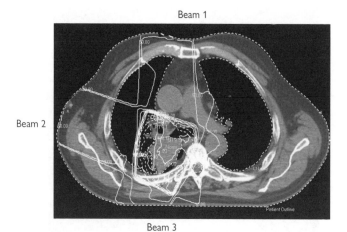

Beam 3

Figure 7.2 Typical radiotherapy treatment plan. The beams of radiation are arranged to ensure that the tumour has an even treatment dose, yet the normal tissues receive as little as possible.

Each radiotherapy session takes about 20 minutes. The actual treatment time is only a minute or two. Most time is taken ensuring that the treatment is correctly and accurately given. When the treatment is actually being given, patients are left alone in the treatment room, although the radiographer can see them through a special window or on a television system.

The side-effects of radiotherapy

Because normal tissues as well as the tumour are being treated by the radiation, side-effects are inevitable. When radiotherapy is given it can have side-effects that are either acute (during or less than 90 days after treatment) and late (more than 90 days after treatment). Late effects are often progressive and, although theoretically reversible, limited effective treatment options exist. This helps explain why the planning process for radiotherapy is rigorous and why so much time is taken to ensure that daily treatment is accurate to reduce these risks.

Common acute side-effects include:

◆ *Cough.* Inflammation of the lung caused by the radiotherapy will often lead to a dry, irritating cough that can be troublesome. Cough suppressants will help and, if severe, the doctor will prescribe steroids such as prednisolone.

◆ *Pain on swallowing.* The oesophagus (gullet) is sensitive to radiation and radiotherapy treatment to the centre of the chest, where lung cancer is commonly situated, will often cause temporary pain and discomfort on eating or swallowing. This comes the week after treatment and subsides over a period of 3–4 weeks. Eating soft foods, not too hot, not too cold, and drugs that line the oesophagus such as Gaviscon™ can help.

◆ *Tiredness.* This is very common during and after radiotherapy treatment and builds up during the course of the treatment. It will usually improve fairly quickly in the first few weeks after stopping treatment. Tiredness associated with cancer and its treatment is poorly researched and understood, but increasingly exercise rehabilitation, rather than rest—the traditional doctor and nurse cure-all—is thought to help.

◆ *Nausea and loss of appetite.* Most patients will notice nausea if large areas of the body are being treated, and some loss of appetite that usually returns.

◆ *Reddening and soreness of the skin.* You should not expect this to be anything other than some pinkness following radiotherapy for lung cancer.

What can be achieved with radiotherapy?

Palliative treatment. It is estimated that at least half of all cancer patients receive radiotherapy at some time during their illness. It is thus the commonest treatment given for lung cancer.

When the objective is palliation, the major symptoms that seem to be helped are:

◆ coughing up blood;

◆ chest pain;

◆ breathlessness caused by collapse of part of the lung;

◆ swelling of the neck or face caused by pressure on large veins in the chest (superior vena caval obstruction).

Palliative radiotherapy can also be used to help the symptoms that result when lung cancer spreads. For example:

◆ pain caused by tumour in a bone;

◆ symptoms caused by tumour in the brain or tumour pressing on a nerve;

◆ tumour in the skin causing an ulcer.

Radiotherapy can relieve symptoms from these problems in 40–85% of patients.

It is not uncommon for some patients to discover by chance that they have lung cancer when they have no symptoms, for example on a routine chest X-ray done before an operation. If the aim of treatment is then purely palliative, and there are no symptoms, then there is no harm in delaying radiotherapy until those symptoms start.

Radical treatment. The days when it was said that no patients could be cured who did not undergo surgery are now over. For smaller tumours when patients are not fit for surgery, radiotherapy will stop at least 40% of tumours <4 cm in size growing within 2 years. Thirty-five per cent of patients with stage I disease will be alive after 5 years, which may be equivalent to surgery given that many of these patients have major medical problems that prevent surgery being done, and from which they die rather than from the cancer. Even with locally advanced inoperable disease, aggressive therapies with combinations of radiotherapy and chemotherapy can result in 15% of patients being alive at 5 years.

Drug therapy for non-small cell lung cancer

Drug therapy for cancer used to be confined to chemotherapy. A rapid increase in our knowledge of the nature of cancer and the ability to design drugs at a molecular level has allowed the development of newer, more targeted agents with some now entering routine clinical use. Chemotherapy is usually drug treatment which tries to kill cancer cells or stop them spreading. Different types of cancer cells and cancers respond to different drugs, so not all chemotherapy is the same.

Chemotherapy

Chemotherapy remains a very important part of the treatment of lung cancer but by itself cannot cure non-small cell lung cancer. Because it can sometimes cause severe side-effects, the potential benefits of treatment (tumour shrinkage, control of symptoms, prolongation of life) must be carefully weighed against the known disadvantages. Over the past two decades there has been a marked increase in the use of chemotherapy. This has occurred as a consequence of two large reviews of all the available clinical trial data by a process called meta-analysis, which showed that chemotherapy prolonged survival in advanced disease. In addition several new anticancer drugs have become available, and we now know that when chemotherapy is combined with other treatments such as radiotherapy there are better outcomes in patients with locally advanced disease.

Like radiotherapy, chemotherapy drugs can stop cancer cells dividing and reproducing themselves. As the drugs are carried in the blood, they can reach cancer cells anywhere in the body. They are also taken up by some healthy cells. Healthy cells can repair the damage caused by chemotherapy, but cancer cells cannot and so they eventually die. Chemotherapy drugs attack cells in a number of different ways—sometimes in the cytoplasm but most commonly in the DNA or nucleus of the cell, where they can stop cells growing and dividing by interfering with cellular processes at different stages of the cell cycle, or life cycle of a cell.

The cell cycle

* **G0 phase (resting stage)**. The cell has not yet started to divide. Cells spend much of their lives in this phase. Depending on the type of cell, G0 can last for a few hours to a few years. When the cell is signalled to reproduce, it moves into the G1 phase.

* **G1 phase**. During this phase, the cell starts making more proteins and growing larger, so the new cells will be of normal size. This phase lasts about 18–30 hours.

* **S phase**. In the S phase, the chromosomes containing the genetic code (DNA) are copied so that both of the new cells formed will have matching

strands of DNA. This phase lasts about 18–20 hours. Antimetabolites, e.g. mitomycin C, work here.

◆ **G2 phase**. In the G2 phase, the cell checks the DNA and prepares to start dividing into two cells. It lasts from 2 to 10 hours.

◆ **M phase (mitosis)**. In this phase, which lasts only 30–60 minutes, the cell actually divides into two new cells. Alkaloids such as vinorelbine and vincristine work here.

Drugs such as cisplatin and cyclophosphamide (an alkylating agent) can work in any part of the cell cycle.

A number of anticancer drugs in common use can have benefits in non-small cell lung cancer. Usually combinations of two drugs are used. Single drugs tend to be given to patients who have already received treatment, or who are more elderly or generally unwell and when there are concerns about tolerance of more aggressive therapy. There is no evidence that giving more than two drugs together improves on the results; rather, they simply add further side-effects. When first tested, chemotherapy drugs are thought of as useful if they can shrink the size of a cancer by more than 50%. This is called the response rate. Most single agent drugs used in the treatment of non-small cell lung cancer have response rates of 15–30% in patients who have had no previous treatment. Using combinations of drugs for treatment, these response rates are 30–50%.

The backbone of chemotherapy for non-small cell lung cancer is currently based on two platinum drugs, either cisplatin or carboplatin. Either drug can be used in combination with drugs such as vinorelbine, gemcitabine, irinotecan, pemetrexed, and the taxanes: docetaxel and paclitaxel.

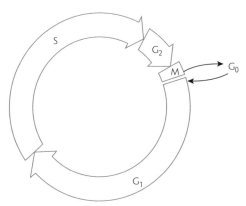

Figure 7.3 The cell cycle.

The drugs most commonly used as single agents in previously untreated patients are gemcitabine and vinorelbine.

Table 7.2 lists commonly used chemotherapy drugs in non-small cell lung cancer, how they are given, and their likely side-effects

How you have chemotherapy. Almost all chemotherapy drugs for lung cancer are given by injection into a vein or through a drip, although there are now some that can be taken as tablets by mouth at home, such as vinorelbine, and more are under development. How you have the drugs—and how often—depends on with which drugs your doctor is treating you. Usually, you have treatment with a combination of two different chemotherapy drugs together. Most often, each chemotherapy treatment is given over 1–3 days. Then you have a rest period of 3 weeks. This allows your body to get over any side-effects. The number of treatments you have depends on:

- which drugs you are having;
- the type of cancer you have;
- whether or not the cancer is responding;
- how your body is coping with the side-effects.

You can have most chemotherapy drugs as an outpatient. So you come in for the day to have treatment and go home afterwards. Your chemotherapy nurse will give you medicines for side-effects to take home in case you need them.

Table 7.2 Common drugs used for non-small cell lung cancer

Drug	Usual duration and schedule for intravenous infusion	Commonest adverse effects
Carboplatin	1 hour every 21 days	Thrombocytopenia, neutropenia, anaemia
Cisplatin	1–2 hours every 21 days, with hydration	Nausea, vomiting, renal impairment, anaemia, neuropathy, tinnitus, hearing loss
Docetaxel	1 hour every 21 days	Neutropenia, fluid retention, neuropathy, alopecia
Gemcitabine	30 minutes every 7 days	Thrombocytopenia, lethargy
Paclitaxel	3 hours every 21 days	Neutropenia, neuropathy, allergic reactions, hair loss
Pemetrexed	10 minutes every 3 weeks, with vitamins	Nausea and tiredness, neutropenia
Irinotecan	30 minutes every 3 weeks	Neutropenia, diarrhoea, sickness, hair loss
Vinorelbine	5–10 minutes every 7 days	Neutropenia, neuropathy, pain during infusion, reddening at infusion site

Some chemotherapy drugs have to be given in hospital; rarely does this mean more than one night in hospital. Usually this is because you have to have them given through a drip over a number of hours.

How many treatments? Most chemotherapy is given for three or four treatments. A full course takes about 3 months. Your doctor will review your progress by monitoring your symptoms and if necessary by checking the size of your cancer on scans and X-rays. It may be very upsetting to be told your treatment is being stopped after only two treatments when you thought you'd have four to six. But your specialist really does have your best interests at heart and will not suggest stopping unless there is no sign of the treatment working or it is causing intolerable side-effects

Side-effects of chemotherapy. There is now an emphasis on making treatment easier to handle with fewer side-effects. Thus not all combinations now require hair loss. Antisickness drugs have considerably improved and are routinely given as prevention. The National Institute for Health and Clinical Excellence gives guidance to doctors as to what treatment should be given and National Cancer Standards dictate how the drugs should be given in the safest way. However, we have not yet reached the stage where chemotherapy has no side-effects, and for some patients they can be life-threatening, in particular, suppression of the immune system leading to what is called febrile neutropenia: febrile (raised temperature), neutropenia (very low white blood cell count). This is a medical emergency and often requires admission to hospital for antibiotics. Other frequent side-effects common to all chemotherapy treatments include:

- tiredness;
- nausea;
- some fluid retention;
- skin changes.

Before each treatment is given, the blood count and often liver and kidney function are checked to ensure that they are adequate to tolerate the toxic effects of the chemotherapy. Sometimes treatment has to be delayed to allow these blood tests, particularly the white cell count, to return to safe levels. These delays do not affect the chances of the treatment working.

Targeted therapies

A better understanding of the mechanisms of disease has resulted in major changes in our approach to cancer therapy. The identification of specific targets within and sometimes unique to cancer cells, rather than normal cells such as receptors or proteins, has allowed the development of new agents. The objective is to identify those things in the tumours that are sufficiently different from normal tissues to be effectively targeted. Targeted drugs have a specific mechanism of action, by contrast to conventional chemotherapy which usually has a non-specific mechanism. In general, targeted therapy refers to the use of biological products, cells, or proteins. These can include hormones, antibodies, targeted small molecules, and vaccines.

Monoclonal antibodies

Modern technology has allowed the production within the laboratory of potentially unlimited quantities of monoclonal antibodies directed against specific targets. There are two major types of monoclonal antibodies. The most common currently used are so-called chimerized/humanized antibodies. These are produced using human sequences of DNA stimulated within a mouse.

Fully human antibodies are produced in specific genetically engineered mice. These mice use human DNA to make human antibodies. The best known monoclonal antibody is Herceptin®, used in the treatment of breast cancer. As yet, monoclonal antibodies have not made a large impact on lung cancer. However, one such monoclonal antibody called cetuximab, which is an antibody against the epidermal growth factor receptor (EGFR), has recently shown an advantage when given in combination with chemotherapy.

Small molecule technology

Small molecule drugs block specific enzyme pathways and growth factor receptors. Protein tyrosine kinase can be one such inhibitor. Small molecule inhibitors of vascular endothelial growth factor and EGFR have recently shown benefit in clinical trials in lung cancer.

Epidermal growth factor receptor inhibitors

The EGFR sits on the surface of many types of cancer cells and there seems to be more of these on cancer cells than on normal cells. These receptors allow the epidermal growth factor to attach to them. When growth factors bind to the receptors, a protein called tyrosine kinase can make chemical signals that tells the cell to grow and divide. Drugs such as erlotinib or gefitinib can attach themselves to the tyrosine kinase protein and this stops chemical signals from being produced which should stop the cell from dividing. Approximately 70–80% of non-small cell lung cancers overexpress this receptor and it is an attractive target for treatment.

These drugs also have the advantage that they are given by tablet, but they can have side-effects.

Interestingly these drugs seem to work best when there is an abnormality in the EGFR, a so-called mutation, in the genetic structure. These mutations tend to be more common in people of Asian descent, women and lifelong non-smokers. An active area of research is to better select patients for any specific treatment by doing special tests in the laboratory known as molecular markers.

Currently these drugs are used when other treatments, largely platinum-based chemotherapy, has failed. There is also some information suggesting that these drugs may reduce the time after chemotherapy with platinum drugs before the cancer progresses or starts to cause further symptoms. It is not yet known whether this treatment actually prolongs overall survival. This at first sight seems a strange concept, but if a drug is given it may result in the same length of life, no matter at what stage of the disease it is given. The rapid development of new drugs means that there are now more choices for treatment. For example, the survival time when gefitininb is prescribed is the same as with further chemotherapy when first-line chemotherapy fails, but the quality of life is better.

Blood supply and cancer

Angiogenesis is the term used to describe the growth of new blood vessels. Cancers need to grow their own blood vessels as they get bigger. Without its own blood supply, a cancer cannot continue to grow. Anti-angiogenesis is the name for treatment to block the development of new blood vessels. This is also a type of biological therapy. The drug thalidomide is a good example of the importance of careful clinical studies with drugs. Thalidomide was first used as an effective antisickness medication in pregnant women. It resulted in a scandal in the 1960s causing birth defects in children, but it is also an anti-angiogenic drug. Unfortunately large trials have not confirmed the initial promise of this drug in the treatment of lung cancer.

Bevacizumab (also called Avastin®) is also an anti-angiogenic monoclonal antibody. It can be used for the treatment of advanced non-small cell lung cancer, in combination with chemotherapy. Studies with this drug have resulted in more than 50% of patients with lung cancer that has spread surviving for more than 12 months. This may not seem much but is a big improvement in the average 3–4-month survival for advanced lung cancer 20 years ago. It reminds us that progress in cancer treatments is not the giant leap forward that we really want but a series of small steps of gradual improvement.

Hormonal therapy

Certain cancers, for example, prostate and breast cancer, are known to be hormonally driven. Unfortunately this is not the case for lung cancer and these drugs do not work.

What is the best treatment for me?

It is important to ask your doctor a number of questions in helping you both to come to a treatment decision. Nowadays you can expect to have the help of a specialist nurse in lung cancer to help you make treatment choices. Furthermore your treatment should have been discussed by a multidisciplinary team. This is made up of all the healthcare staff involved in your care—includings cancer nurses and all the main consultants, including radiologists, radiotherapists, surgeons, and physicians. General questions should be:

- Who should I contact if I am worried?
- What help is available for my family?
- What patient support groups are there locally?
- How quickly will the treatment start?

- What will the treatment be like and how long will it take?
- Will there be side-effects and what can I do about them?
- Is my surgeon a specialist in my form of cancer?
- Who prescribes the chemotherapy?
- Who will give the chemotherapy?
- Can I have the chemotherapy in my local hospital?
- Can I have my surgery, radiotherapy, or chemotherapy more quickly if I have them outside normal office hours?
- How quickly will the treatment start?

Then some more specific questions need to be asked, for example:

- Why do I need treatment?
- Are there alternative treatments?
- Should I take special precautions during treatment?
- What are the aims of treatment?
- How long will the treatment go on for?
- What are the chances it will benefit me?
- Is the treatment part of a trial or can I access a trial in another centre?

Treatment by stage

Stage 0 (carcinoma *in situ*)

It is very rare to diagnose lung cancer at such a very early stage. It would only usually be found by accident (if you were having investigations for something else). Normal treatment is to remove a small part of the lung in an operation:

1. Segmental or wedge resection (operation).
2. Occasionally photodynamic therapy may be advised.

Stage I: non-small cell lung cancer

For this stage you would preferably have surgery, but more lung tissue removed than for stage 0. The most likely operation is a lobectomy, in which part of the lung and some of the lymph nodes are removed. A further option if you can't have an operation for other health reasons (for example there is not enough spare heart or lung capacity) is radical radiotherapy. A very few patients are also treated by radiofrequency ablation (page 91).

Treatment of stage I non-small cell lung cancer may thus include the following:

- Surgery (wedge resection, segmental resection, or lobectomy).
- External beam radiotherapy (for patients who cannot have surgery or choose not to have surgery).

- Surgery followed by chemotherapy.
- Radiofrequency ablation.

Stage II: non-small cell lung cancer

For stage II lung cancer you will probably be offered lobectomy or pneumonectomy. If the cancer is completely removed your specialist may suggest chemotherapy to try to reduce the risk of the cancer returning. Again, if you cannot have an operation you may be offered radiotherapy.

Treatment of stage II non-small cell lung cancer may include the following:

- Surgery (wedge resection, segmental resection, lobectomy, or pneumonectomy).
- External beam radiotherapy (for patients who cannot have surgery or choose not to have surgery).
- Surgery followed by chemotherapy, with or without other treatments.

Stages IIIA and IIIB: non-small cell lung cancer

For stage III lung cancer, fewer patients are able to have an operation, because the whole lung may need to be removed. In addition, the cancer can be too close to your heart or major blood vessels to operate safely. Treatment can be chemotherapy and then surgery, chemotherapy and radiotherapy, rarely chemotherapy, radiotherapy, and surgery.

Treatment of stage IIIA non-small cell lung cancer may include the following:

- Surgery with or without radiation therapy.
- External beam radiotherapy alone.
- Chemotherapy combined with other treatments.
- Combinations of surgery, chemotherapy, radiotherapy.

Treatment of stage IIIB non-small cell lung cancer may include the following:

- External radiation therapy alone.
- Chemotherapy combined with external radiation therapy.
- Chemotherapy combined with external radiation therapy, followed by surgery.
- Chemotherapy alone.
- Clinical trial of new ways of giving radiation therapy.
- Clinical trial of new combinations of treatments.

Stage IV: non-small cell lung cancer

Unfortunately once the cancer has spread there is no cure and the objective of treatment is to help the symptoms. Radiotherapy can help symptoms, as can internal radiotherapy (brachytherapy), laser treatment, using a rigid tube (a stent to keep the airway open), chemotherapy, and immunotherapy.

Treatment of stage IV non-small cell lung cancer may include the following:

◆ Watchful waiting until symptoms develop.

◆ External radiation therapy as palliative therapy, to relieve pain and other symptoms and improve the quality of life.

◆ Chemotherapy with or without antibody therapy.

◆ Laser therapy and/or internal radiation therapy.

◆ A clinical trial of chemotherapy with or without biological therapies.

Maintenance treatment

Once the cancer is under control or in remission or has been completely removed, a common question is what can be done to keep it either away or at bay. Chapter 13 deals with ways in which patients can help themselves but there are also new drugs that may help. The EGFR inhibitor erlotinib is being tested after surgery to see if it can improve overall survival. There is already information showing that it can prolong the time before the cancer progresses after initial chemotherapy. The hope is that it will prolong the overall survival but this is not yet known.

Treatment at relapse

Ten years ago many patients with lung cancer received no treatment at all. With the rapid increase of available drugs it is now quite common for patients to receive not only a second treatment, but sometimes third or fourth treatments, if their general health permits and they wish to continue with treatment.

Common second-line and further treatments include, after failure of chemotherapy:

◆ Second-line chemotherapy with drugs such as docetaxel and pemetrexed.

◆ EGFR inhibitors such as erlotinib.

◆ Palliative radiotherapy to areas causing symptoms.

◆ Best supportive care alone.

◆ Local palliative therapies (see page 89).

8

Treatment of small cell lung cancer

 Key points

- Small cell lung cancer can grow and spread aggressively.
- Chemotherapy is the major treatment for small cell lung cancer.
- Radiotherapy is given to the lungs of patients with disease confined within the chest.

Radiotherapy is given to the brain when there is a good response to chemotherapy.

In contrast to other types of lung cancer where surgery is the mainstay of treatment, chemotherapy and radiotherapy are the major treatments used. This is because small cell lung cancer can grow and spread rapidly. Less than 1% of patients receive surgery, usually as part of investigation of a small nodule within the lung where it is removed to make a diagnosis. For these patients surgery should always be followed by chemotherapy. The prognosis is that about half of this unusual group of patients will survive.

The staging of small cell lung cancer is simplified to reflect treatment options and prognosis. It is divided into limited disease, which in practical terms means that the disease is suitable for radiotherapy and extensive disease (see page 43). About 30% of patients present with limited disease. The other major prognostic factor is how fit patients are. Perhaps not surprisingly the best results are in patients who are fit (see the performance status boxes in Chapter 6, pages 54 and 55) and with limited disease. The disease is, however, usually characterized by good initial response to treatment but often rapid relapse and the overall 5-year survival rate is no more than 5–10%.

Chemotherapy
Limited disease

When chemotherapy is given initially it is called first-line therapy. Approximately 80% of patients with limited disease will respond to chemotherapy. When single drugs are used the response rate (page 69) is about 40%. However, single drugs rarely cause complete disappearance of tumour, and thus it has become standard practice to use combinations of drugs. The most common combination of drugs in use is cisplatin or its sister drug carboplatin with etoposide (Table 8.1). Clinical trials have not shown advantage to adding a third drug, only increased side-effects. Other drugs used at presentation include doxorubicin, cyclophosphamide, vincristine and irinotecan. Four to six courses or cycles of treatment are commonly given depending on how the tumour responds to treatment and importantly how the treatment is tolerated.

Extensive disease

A more common presentation in 60–70% of cases is with extensive disease. The drugs used are the same as those for the treatment of limited disease. The chance of the cancer shrinking with combinations of drugs is about 60% in patients with extensive disease. There is no good evidence that more than three or four courses of treatment are necessary, particularly when patients are frail.

These treatments are given by a combination of drips into the vein and tablets. All anticancer drugs have side-effects. In particular, all combinations of treatment for small cell lung cancer cause hair loss, and may cause sickness which can be prevented at least in part by modern anti-sickness drugs. Tiredness and lethargy are common to most drugs used for this condition. All chemotherapy drugs can suppress the immune system whether given by drip or tablet, and if a high temperature develops urgent admission to hospital may be needed. Selection for chemotherapy, and administration by whom, is now carefully regulated and reviewed under national cancer standards.

It is important to remember that not everyone will have all of these side-effects and you can expect to be given written information not only about your treatment but also what to do if you become unwell.

Second-line treatments

Sadly the disease comes back or relapses in the majority of patients after treatment. Treatment is then termed second-line. The outlook can be very poor at

Table 8.1 Common drugs used for small cell lung cancer

Drug	Usual duration and schedule for intravenous infusion	Commonest adverse effects
Carboplatin	1 hour every 21 days	Thrombocytopenia, neutropenia, anaemia
Cisplatin	1–2 hours every 21 days, with hydration	Nausea, vomiting, renal impairment, anaemia, neuropathy, tinnitus, hearing loss
Etoposide	1 hour daily for 3 days every 21 days	Neutropenia, hair loss

this stage. If there has been less than 3 months between completing first-line treatment and relapse, the disease is unlikely to respond to chemotherapy and such treatment is rarely advised. If more than 3 months occurs before relapse and patients remain fit for treatment, then second-line treatment is usually considered. The chance of responding to treatment is 45–50%, but treatment usually works for a shorter duration than with first-line therapies. Treatment is usually given with combinations of two to three drugs. The drugs used are usually different from those used first time, in case the tumour has developed resistance to the initial therapies. One commonly used combination is vincristine, adriamycin and cyclophosphamide.

Radiotherapy
Chest radiotherapy

The major advance in the treatment of small cell lung cancer in the last 30 years is the more widespread use of radiotherapy. Traditionally radiotherapy to the chest has been given at completion of chemotherapy for patients with limited disease who respond well to chemotherapy. This treatment not only can delay the return of the cancer, but also improve the overall cure rate by 5%. In many different types of cancers treated with radiotherapy it has become clear that the results are improved by giving chemotherapy at the same time or concurrently with radiotherapy. Such treatment is now standard care for locally advanced cancers of the cervix, head and neck, and oesophagus (gullet). More recent studies have looked at giving radiotherapy with chemotherapy earlier in the treatment of small cell lung cancer. For very fit patients with limited disease, concurrent treatment improves the 2-year survival rate by a further 5% compared with giving the radiotherapy at the end of chemotherapy. Usually radiotherapy is given once daily, Monday to Friday. For small cell lung cancer patients there may be an advantage for that treatment to be given twice daily with chemotherapy.

Radiotherapy to the brain

The second advance with radiotherapy was the discovery that giving treatment to the brain after chemotherapy improved survival. The delicate structures of our brains are protected by a blood–brain barrier which stops chemicals transferring from the bloodstream into the fluids that bathe our brains. Usually this is helpful in protecting us from all the unpleasant chemicals in the environment, but in this situation it also prevents chemotherapy drugs from entering the brain. For patients who survive for more than 2 years after treatment, one of the commonest places the cancer can recur is within the brain. This causes very unpleasant symptoms such as weakness of limbs, headaches, and confusion. Treatment in this situation has only a limited benefit and the prognosis is poor. Prophylactic cranial irradiation is the term used for giving radiotherapy at the end of chemotherapy to try to prevent the development of cancer spread to the brain. Initially this treatment was just given to patients with limited disease who responded well to chemotherapy. This treatment improves the survival rates at

3 years by nearly 6% and reduces the incidence of brain metastases by half. More recent research has shown that this treatment can also benefit patients with extensive disease who respond well to chemotherapy, again reducing the incidence of symptomatic brain metastases and improving survival. Treatment is usually given in 10 daily treatments over 2 weeks. Side-effects include headache, tiredness and either hair loss, or a delay in re-growth of hair when chemotherapy has been given previously. Initially there was concern that radiotherapy may cause problems with brain function such as concentration, memory, and spatial awareness. More recent trials have shown that so long as the radiation dose is kept at relatively modest levels these symptoms are no more likely in patients who undergo radiotherapy compared with those treated with chemotherapy alone.

Palliative radiotherapy

Radiotherapy can also be given to help symptoms just as for non-small cell lung cancer. Thus, often one or two treatments can help with symptoms such as coughing up blood, or pain from spread of cancer to the bones (page 99).

Newer treatments

Systemic chemotherapy has not really improved in small cell lung cancer in the last 30 years. Overall results have probably improved because of improvements in the organization of services rather than because of the treatments themselves. Thus more patients have biopsy samples taken to confirm the diagnosis, and team-working means that all lung cancer patients will be treated by specialists in lung cancer treatment. The results remain disappointing and new approaches and treatments are urgently required.

Over the last few years our understanding of the biology of cancer has developed rapidly. The aim is to find features unique to tumour cells that can be targeted rather than the much more broad attack of chemotherapy drugs that

Table 8.2 Recommendations for the more common situations

Stage	Good performance status (fit)	Poor performance status (unfit)
Limited	4–6 cycles chemotherapy. Either concurrent or sequential chest radiotherapy. Prophylactic cranial irradiation.	4–6 cycles chemotherapy. Possible sequential chest radiotherapy and prophylactic cranial irradiation in responders if condition allows.
Extensive	3 or 4 cycles chemotherapy, two drugs. Prophylactic cranial irradiation in responders.	Treatment individualized. Either 3 or 4 cycles chemotherapy or supportive care alone.

cause damage to normal as well as abnormal cells. At present this approach has been much more fruitful in non-small cell than in small cell lung cancer.

Current recommendations for treatment

Where the tumour is small, usually in the outer part of the lung and there is no sign of spread on scans, an operation to remove the tumour is indicated followed by six courses of chemotherapy and then prophylactic cranial irradiation (Table 8.2).

Results of treatment

Untreated, the prognosis of this condition is very poor with an average survival of 4 months for limited and 2 months for extensive disease respectively. With treatment the average survival is 18 months for limited and 9 months for extensive disease. In spite of these figures up to 10% of cases, who are usually fit patients with limited disease, are cured of their cancer and at least 30% of patients treated with chemotherapy and radiotherapy for limited disease will be alive after 2 years.

9

Treatment of other lung tumours

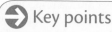 Key points

- Mesothelioma is caused by exposure to asbestos.
- There is a current epidemic of mesothelioma.
- Treatment of mesothelioma is largely to control the symptoms.

Mesothelioma

Mesothelioma is a tumour that develops in the lining of the lung known as the pleura. At the turn of the twentieth century this cancer was virtually unheard of. At the moment there is an epidemic of this tumour due to a clear-cut relationship to previous asbestos exposure.

The pleura wraps itself around the lung and covers the inside of the chest wall. It is made up of a thin inner lining (visceral pleura) and a thicker outer lining (parietal pleura). The space between the two layers of the pleura is called the pleural cavity. The two layers are normally in contact bar a small amount of pleural fluid to provide lubrication as the surfaces move as the lung contracts and expands with breathing. When mesothelioma develops in the pleura (pleural mesothelioma), the delicate membranes thicken and may press inwards on the lung. Fluid may also collect between the two layers of the pleura: this is known as a pleural effusion. A similar lining is found in the abdomen and is called the peritoneum. Mesotheliomas can also occur in the peritoneum but are less common. Rather than starting in the abdomen, more commonly mesothelioma spreads from the chest cavity through the diaphragm into the abdomen.

Who gets mesothelioma?

Virtually all cases of mesothelioma are caused by exposure to asbestos. Asbestos is a natural mineral, mined from rock found in many countries. Asbestos is in many ways an ideal product for builders. It is made up of tiny fibres that are as strong as steel but can be woven like cotton and are highly resistant to heat and chemicals. It thus found its way into many construction and insulation materials in common use after the Second World War. When asbestos is disturbed or damaged, it releases tiny fibres that can be breathed into the lungs. Asbestos fibres are very fine and, when breathed in, they can make their way into the smallest airways of the lung, so they cannot be breathed or coughed out. Once the fibres are in the lungs, the body's defence mechanism tries to break them down and remove them, which leads to an inflammation in the lung tissue.

The asbestos fibres can also penetrate through the lung tissue to settle in the pleura. Over many years this constant irritation to the lungs can cause mesothelioma or other lung diseases called asbestosis to develop. Asbestos fibres can also be swallowed, and some of the fibres can stick in the digestive system. They can then move into the peritoneum where again they cause inflammation that can lead to mesothelioma. During the 1960s the first definite link between mesothelioma and asbestos was made.

The people most likely to have been exposed to asbestos include:

- construction workers;
- plumbers;
- electricians;
- boilermakers;
- shipbuilders;
- demolition workers;
- people who worked in other places where asbestos was present; and
- those who lived near to asbestos factories.

Family members of people who worked with asbestos and brought the dust home on their clothes have also sometimes developed mesothelioma. Washing the clothes released the asbestos fibres into the air to be inhaled.

What causes mesothelioma?

There are three types of asbestos: blue, brown and white. Blue and brown asbestos are the types most commonly linked with mesothelioma. They are now very rarely used and cannot be imported into the UK. Originally, white asbestos was thought not to be dangerous but recent studies have shown that it may also be harmful.

In the 1980s, imports of blue and brown asbestos into the UK were stopped, and in 1999 importing and use of all types of asbestos was banned. However, as mesothelioma develops so slowly, it is estimated that by 2015 about 3,000 people will be diagnosed in the UK with mesothelioma each year. The number of people who develop mesothelioma will then start to reduce each year.

Mesothelioma does not usually develop until many years after exposure to asbestos. This is called the latent period and can take any time from 10 to 60 years, although the average is about 30–40 years.

Occasionally, mesothelioma develops in people who have never been exposed to asbestos. Other causes of this disease are not understood, but in rare cases the development of mesothelioma has been linked to exposure to radiation.

Smoking by itself does not increase the risk of developing mesothelioma. However, for those exposed to asbestos, smoking increases the risk of developing mesothelioma many fold. It is also thought that exposure to other building materials such as fibreglass does not increase the risk.

Symptoms of mesothelioma

Mesothelioma often starts as a lot of tiny lumps (nodules) in the pleura, which may not show up on scans or X-rays until they are quite large. The main symptoms of pleural mesothelioma are breathlessness and chest pain, followed by tiredness and general weakness. The breathlessness is caused by either the lining of the lung being unable to expand with each breath and thus constricting the lungs, or by a build-up of fluid between the two linings of the lung (a pleural effusion). Chest X-rays will show the fluid on the lung and can show other evidence of exposure to asbestos such as changes within the lung fields themselves: in severe cases due to asbestosis (a condition of the lung where it becomes densely scarred) or more commonly speckled deposits of calcium on the outside of the lungs known as pleural plaques. A computed tomography (CT) scan will also show the fluid, thickening of the lining of the lung and may show evidence of spread to local lymph nodes or other organs.

The diagnosis is made by taking a biopsy from the lining of the lung, most commonly either by CT-guided biopsy or thoracoscopy (see page 96).

Treatment of mesothelioma

Surgery

Only a very few patients with very localized mesothelioma can have an operation. Surgery may involve removing part, or all, of the pleura and the lung tissue close to it. This is known as pleurectomy. Sometimes the pleura, diaphragm, and the whole lung on the affected side are removed as well as the tumour. This operation is known as extra-pleural pneumonectomy. This operation is usually done after chemotherapy and is followed by radiotherapy. Such surgery causes considerable morbidity and is very controversial. Clinical trials are ongoing, questioning whether such a massive operation really alters either the quality or quantity of life of patients since the tumour invariably recurs in spite of the surgery.

More commonly the intent of surgical procedures is palliative, that is to relieve symptoms, for example by stopping the pleural fluid re-accumulating.

Chest tube drainage (page 94) and pleurodesis is the most common form of palliative surgical treatment. The build-up of fluid or pleural effusions can be persistent and often recurs rapidly and sometimes repeatedly following initial drainage of the fluid (known as thoracocentesis). In order to stop the fluid re-accumulating, the pleural space can be sealed. This is done by using agents that make an inflammatory reaction between the two linings of the lung after the fluid has been drained to make them stick together. Commonly used drugs include talc slurry, tetracycline, or other sclerosing agents, all of which produce adhesion. Typical surgical approaches to pleurodesis include the following.

Surgical approaches to mesothelioma

- **Thoracoscopy** and **Pleurodesis** is done in conjunction with video assisted thoracoscopy (VATS) using a powdered form of talc known as talc slurry. Both this and chest tube drainage and pleurodesis will be only effective if there is no tumour encasing the lung which restricts its expansion.

- **Pleuroperitoneal shunt** plays a limited role in palliation for several reasons. It involves placement of a catheter run under the skin from the pleural to the peritoneal cavity. Commonly the catheter blocks and there is a considerable risk of seeding of the tumour into the abdominal cavity.

- **Pleurectomy**, used as a palliative procedure, may be performed where more extensive surgery is not an option. In these cases, it is understood that all visible or gross tumour will not be removed. It is considered the most effective means of controlling pleural effusion in cases where the lung's expansion is restricted by disease.

Radiotherapy

Radiotherapy can sometimes shrink or reduce the size of mesothelioma. This can help with symptoms like pain and discomfort, or breathlessness. Usually no more than ten daily treatments are given over 2 weeks. Radiotherapy may also be given to the chest wall at the place where a biopsy has been done or a drainage tube has been inserted. In this situation, the radiotherapy prevents the tumour from growing out through the scar. Between one and three treatments are given to each biopsy site.

Chemotherapy

Chemotherapy may be used to achieve different goals, depending on the stage of the cancer at the time of diagnosis and the age and health of the patient. Chemotherapy for mesothelioma is not considered 'curative'. As with non-small cell lung cancer, in a few cases chemotherapy may be used:

- to shrink tumours prior to other treatments, such as surgery (this is called neoadjuvant chemotherapy);

- to destroy microscopic disease which may remain after surgery (this is called adjuvant chemotherapy);

- for palliation, that is to control the cancer by stopping its spread or slowing its growth—by so doing, symptoms such as pain and breathlessness may be relieved.

Pemetrexed (Alimta®) is a multi-targeted anti-folate drug normally given with cisplatin or carboplatin, and is currently considered the most effective treatment for mesothelioma patients who are not surgical candidates. The side-effects and importantly the risk of death due to the chemotherapy are reduced by the use of vitamin supplements. Thus vitamin B_{12} supplements given by injection into the muscle and oral tablets of folic acid are started in the week prior to treatment. Additionally, oral steroids, given before and after treatment, reduce the risk of skin rash and some other possible side-effects including sickness.

Pemetrexed and cisplatin are usually given intravenously as an outpatient once every 21 days. The treatment involves a 10-minute intravenous drip of pemetrexed, followed by a 2-hour infusion of cisplatin, with some extra fluid for hydration to prevent possible kidney damage caused by the cisplatin. The overall treatment takes about 6 hours. Usually 4–6 cycles of treatment are given dependent on overall response to the treatment. This will include any possible shrinkage of the tumour on scans or X-rays, the effect on symptoms of the disease, and any side-effects that might be experienced.

Side-effects of pemetrexed/cisplatin are usually mild to moderate for most mesothelioma patients, and include nausea, vomiting, and fatigue. For some patients, however, side-effects may be more debilitating, and this may require a decrease in doses of the drugs or even stopping treatment.

Other drugs are now less commonly used in mesothelioma but vinorelbine can be used for palliative benefit when pemetrexed combinations have stopped working. Other drugs used include raltitrexed and gemcitabine, both usually given with cisplatin.

Outlook

The prognosis for mesothelioma is poor and average survival is only between 11 and 14 months.

Compensation

Because of the clear association with asbestos, mesothelioma is thought of legally as an occupational disease. You should be able to claim for compensation from the government as a result. If you have mesothelioma and it can be proved that someone else was responsible for your asbestos exposure, it may be possible to take legal action to claim additional compensation. Legal action taken against former employers is usually dealt with through employers' insurance companies. Legal action may still be possible even as commonly occurs when the employer no longer exists, provided the employer's insurance company can still be traced.

Other rare tumours of the lung

A well as the common types of lung cancer there are several rare tumours that may develop in the lungs. Although for most types of lung cancer there are treatment guidelines based on clinical trial evidence where treatments have been tested, sometimes on thousands of patients, the rarity of these conditions means that there is often limited information about what is the best treatment.

Carcinoid

This is a rare tumour accounting for up to 2.5% of all lung tumours. It is noted for usually following a benign course. Bronchial carcinoids belong to a group of growths called neuroendocrine tumours. Neuorendocrine tumours start in neuroendocrine cells, which are special types of nerve cells that can produce hormones. Hormones control many of the body's functions by controlling the levels of particular chemicals and fluids in the body, and help us respond to changes in our environment. Neuroendocrine tumours range from the relatively benign bronchial carcinoid at one end of the spectrum to the very aggressive small cell carcinoma (see Chapter 8). A group of tumours with intermediate aggressive potential are called atypical carcinoids. Since they come from cells that can make hormones, these tumours often make and secrete chemicals which can cause symptoms such as facial flushing, weakness, diarrhoea, and wheezing. Bronchial carcinoids are not associated with smoking.

Classical carcinoid

The classic or typical bronchial carcinoid is the least aggressive. These tumours are usually well defined, smaller than 2.5 cm in diameter, and located centrally within the main airways. Bronchial carcinoids affect relatively young patients, and usually occur in women. The female:male ratio is 10:1. Only 3% of typical carcinoid tumours spread to sites other than the regional lymph nodes. They are best treated where possible by surgical removal. The prognosis of these tumours is excellent with a 5-year survival rate of 94%. Involvement of regional lymph nodes reduces this survival rate to 71%; however, excellent results may still be achieved with treatment, and the presence of nodal disease does not necessarily stop surgery being performed.

Atypical carcinoid

Atypical carcinoids account for 25% of lung carcinoid tumours. These are more aggressive than typical carcinoids, and usually affect relatively older men. Atypical carcinoids are larger than other carcinoid tumours at presentation, and they tend to occur in the periphery of the lung. Since they are more aggressive, spread to regional lymph nodes is more common, occurring in as many as 50% of patients. Distant spread or metastases to the liver, bone, and brain are seen in one-third of patients. Often these cancers are multiple. Patients with atypical carcinoids have a worse prognosis, with a 5-year survival rate of 57%.

Large cell neuroendocrine carcinoma

Large cell neuroendocrine carcinoma of the lung is a newly recognized entity. This disease is distinct from small cell carcinoma and is associated with a poorer prognosis. The clinical features and optimal treatment of a large cell carcinoma have not yet been established.

Tracheal cancer

The trachea is the main airway leading down into the lungs (see Figure 5.2, page 37). Tracheal cancers occur rarely, accounting for less than 1% of all malignancies. Eighty per cent of all primary tumours of the trachea are malignant. The most common presentation is with wheeze, or as an emergency with obstruction of the trachea. The average length of the adult trachea is 11 cm and it is made up of 18–22 cartilaginous rings, with approximately two rings per centimetre. Surgical resection if possible is the mode of treatment with the best hope for cure. However, the number of cartilaginous rings that can safely be removed is limited to two or three. Radiotherapy can be offered if surgery is not possible. Chemotherapy can also be given less commonly after initial treatment with surgery, radiotherapy, or both. Laser treatment may be performed for relief of symptoms by debulking the tumour and improving the diameter of the airway.

Sarcoma

These are tumours of the supportive structures in the lungs. Their behaviour varies from very slow growing, when spread to other organs is unusual, to highly aggressive rapidly spreading tumours. Treatment is by surgery wherever possible, or by radiotherapy. Chemotherapy is only of use in aggressive tumours.

Lymphomas

Tumours arising from lymph glands are called lymphomas and include Hodgkin's disease and non-Hodgkin's lymphoma. These may involve and indeed rarely even start in the lungs. They should not be regarded as primary lung cancers. They often respond well to non-surgical treatments and in some cases can be cured by combinations of chemotherapy, modern targeted antibody treatments, and radiotherapy.

Secondary tumours

Cancer that spreads from another part of the body to the lungs is very common and should not be regarded as a lung cancer or a new tumour. It is called secondary cancer or metastasis. Treatment depends on where the cancer originally developed and came from.

10

Other methods of treatment

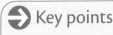 Key points

- There are a number of treatments aimed at destroying cancer locally.
- They are not routine practice and are used in very carefully selected cases, usually in specialist centres.

Despite huge developments in our knowledge of cancer, treatment for lung cancer remains firmly rooted in surgery, radiotherapy, and chemotherapy. Newer, more cancer-targeted agents are making some inroads into the palliative treatments of non-small cell lung cancer, but new approaches continue to be needed. All of the following approaches have their pros and cons and none is widely available.

Hyperthermia

Scientists have known for many years that cancer cells seem to be more sensitive to heat than normal ones. If a tumour is heated up to 41–43°C (normal body temperature is 37°C, then cancer cells are more likely to be killed or seriously damaged than normal cells. As a cancer grows it outstrips its blood supply. Those cancer cells in the middle of the tumour tend to be in an acidic environment and have low oxygen levels. These cells seem to be most resistant to radiotherapy and chemotherapy treatments and potentially most sensitive to hyperthermia. At one time, hyperthermia was used quite extensively but is now rarely used. This is because of the practical difficulties in actually heating tumours to the high temperatures required. Nowadays hyperthermia is largely confined to treating tumours in limbs where it is possible and feasible to provide enough heat at the high temperatures required rather than to heat whole patients for many hours. Heating the whole body to high temperatures puts severe, potentially fatal strains on the heart, lungs, and blood vessels.

Internal irradiation or brachytherapy

Radiotherapy is most commonly given by external beam outside the body. Radiotherapy sources can, however, be implanted inside the body so that they are in contact with a tumour, thus delivering a high dose of radiation directly to the tumour. This technique has been used for many years for patients with cervical cancer and is called brachytherapy. Modern machines called micro-selectrons now allow this treatment to be given into the airways of patients with lung cancer. Its major use is therefore in treating tracheal tumours and tumours blocking main airways, i.e. those places that are potentially accessible for this treatment. Clinical trials have shown that standard external beam radio-therapy treatment gives better survival and symptom control rates as a first palliative treatment. As a result, brachytherapy is now largely used when external beam radiotherapy has failed and for symptom relief.

The treatment is done by passing a thin tube into the airway using the flexible bronchoscope (page 40). The tumour position is marked using X-rays on this tube which is visible on a chest X-ray. The micro-selectron is then programmed to automatically pass the radioactive sources to the site of the tumour. Treatment takes about 20 minutes and can be done as a day case.

Laser treatment

The most simple use of lasers is to cut a passage through a tumour that is block-ing a major airway. It takes about 1 hour and the laser light is passed though a flexible bronchoscope. Unfortunately efficacy of this treatment usually only lasts a short while and thus it usually has to be repeated after a few weeks. As a result, laser treatment is often combined with other treatments such as radio-therapy.

Photodynamic therapy (PDT)

Certain naturally occurring chemicals called haematoporphyrins bind better to, and for longer to, tumour cells than normal cells. Normally these chemicals are harmless but when exposed to red light a chemical reaction can occur and kill the cell. Lasers can produce powerful light sources of different colours or frequencies including red light which can activate the haematoporphyrin.

These reactions may allow us to detect cancers at an earlier stage. Many smok-ers have precancerous changes in the lining of their lungs that can be detectable by this method. In turn this may also give an opportunity to treat these changes before they turn malignant. Just as important is that these precancerous changes can reverse themselves if the patient stops smoking.

Photodynamic therapy can also be used to treat very early cancers. The depth of a tumour that can be treated by this technique is limited as PDT only pen-etrates into tissue to a depth of about 0.5 to 1 cm (about ¼ inch). It is thus best for tumours of the lining of the airway (endobronchial). PDT can control early endobronchial cancer in about three-quarters of patients treated. Surgery remains the preferred treatment where possible. The major side-effect of PDT is photosensitivity, or sensitivity to light. Most people find this inconvenient, but not intolerable. The photosensitizing drug currently used for PDT stays in the skin for about 4–6 weeks. During this time period, care must be taken to prevent too much exposure to bright lights, including sunlight. As the diseased tissue breaks down, it causes inflammation which can cause mild pain. A third side-effect of PDT for lung cancer is shortness of breath. This occurs from fluid build-up in the lungs after PDT.

Radiofrequency ablation (RFA)

This is based on the principle of destroying tumours with high energy radio-waves. This treatment is called 'percutaneous radiofrequency ablation' or RFA. Ablation means destroying. Percutaneous means 'through the skin'. A needle electrode is placed through the skin and into the lung tumour directed by a computed tomography (CT) scan. Radiowaves pass through the needle and can heat the cancer cells in an attempt to destroy them.

Radiofrequency ablation seems to work best for small, early lung cancers that are 3 cm across or less and is increasingly used to treat other cancers that have spread from elsewhere into the lung. The most common complication of RFA is air getting into the chest cavity (pneumothorax). Clinical trials have not yet been done to compare this treatment with standard surgery or radiotherapy. RFA tends to be used if patients cannot have surgery for other health reasons.

Cryotherapy

In this technique a probe is inserted usually through a rigid bronchoscope under general anaesthetic. The tumour is visualized directly and the probe freezes and thaws the tumour, causing it to be destroyed. It can improve the diameter of the airway and thus unblock the major airways. Currently it is used when other treatments have failed, purely for symptom relief.

11

Treatment of the symptoms and complications of lung cancer

Many patients will have symptoms from their lung cancer when they first see their doctor, or will likely develop symptoms later if the tumour is not controlled. This section outlines some of the problems that can arise and discusses how they are treated, although it is important to remember that many patients will develop only a few of these symptoms. Of course, the best treatment for any symptom is to get rid of the underlying cause—the cancer. However, even if this is not possible for some patients, there are many ways in which symptoms can be reduced to improve quality of life.

Lung collapse

Lung cancers, because they grow in the main airways, may obstruct the air passages supplying part or all of a lung (Figure 11.1). The severity of symptoms produced will depend on the amount of lung that is affected. Early symptoms include cough, haemoptysis (coughing up blood), shortness of breath on exertion, and wheezing. If the obstruction becomes complete, a persistent cough, with or without blood in the sputum, may develop and chest discomfort, shortness of breath, and wheeze may become more severe. Infection often develops in the collapsed part of the lung and this will cause fevers and chills, reduction in appetite, weight loss, and symptoms of feeling generally tired and unwell. This infection should be treated with antibiotics regardless of other therapies.

Ideally, treatment is given to shrink the tumour so that the blockage is removed. Radiotherapy (page 64) can be very effective, although it should be remembered that it is usually not possible to use radiotherapy more than once or twice, as it will cause unacceptable damage to the normal tissues in the chest. Chemotherapy (page 68) can be helpful in some tumours although the side-effects of treatment must be weighed carefully against the benefits in non-small cell lung cancer.

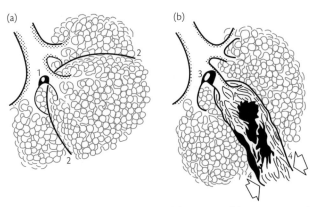

Figure 11.1 Collapse of a segment of the lung. (a) A tumour (1) starts to grow in the airway supplying a segment of lung that is bordered by fibrous bands (2). (b) The tumour (3) grows and nearly completely blocks the airway to the segment. This results in collapse (arrows) of the fibrous borders (4) of the segment and infection.

Other treatments are given into the airway directly. These techniques are only available in some hospitals and some are described in Chapter 10.

If it is not possible to give treatment to remove the blockage, then treatment should be directed at removing troublesome symptoms such as cough (page 103), infection, and pain (page 103).

Venous obstruction: superior vena caval obstruction

A large tumour growing in the centre of the chest may press on the major veins as they are about to enter the heart (Figure 11.2). This large vein (the superior vena cava) drains blood from the head, neck, arms, and upper chest. Any significant pressure on the vein will slow down the blood drainage and all the veins in the area that should be drained will become overfull and distended. This results in swelling of the face, neck, and upper chest and arms. Veins in these areas frequently become more visible than normal. A headache on stooping down due to change in the blood flow to the brain is a common first symptom.

The first treatment given is usually an attempt at placing a tube called a stent in the superior vena cava (SVC) to allow blood to flow again. SVC stenting is done without surgery and a general anaesthetic, and is performed in the X-ray department. An interventional radiologist can perform the entire procedure through a tube (intravenous cannula) inserted into a vein in the groin or neck, after numbing the area with local anaesthetic. At the end, when the cannula is removed, stitches are not required. The procedure usually takes about an hour

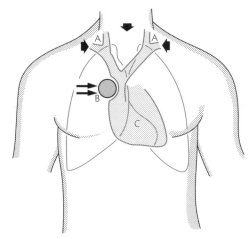

Figure 11.2 Superior vena caval obstruction. The blood from the neck and arms drains into the main veins in the chest (short arrows and A). A tumour (B) pressing on the main vein (the superior vena cava) before it enters the heart (C) will block the blood vessel, causing back pressure and swelling of the neck, arms, and face.

to complete. The symptoms of venous obstruction commonly resolve rapidly in a few days. There are small risks (1%) of bleeding and the stent can block at a later date, so it is common for blood-thinning drugs (anticoagulants) to be prescribed.

Further treatment to control the cancer, such as radiotherapy or chemotherapy, may then be advised. Steroids may also be used to try to reduce the amount of oedema and swelling. If radiotherapy has been used and cannot be repeated, chemotherapy and/or steroids may help reduce the pressure on the superior vena cava.

Pleural effusion

What is it?

A pleural effusion is a collection of fluid between the chest wall and the lung. It typically develops between the two linings of the lung (pleura). Because the fluid compresses the lung it will cause shortness of breath as it gets larger (Figure 11.3).

How can it be dealt with?

It is a relatively simple procedure to remove the fluid from a pleural effusion that has become large enough to cause troublesome breathlessness. For patients who have not had problems from the effusion before, it may be enough to push

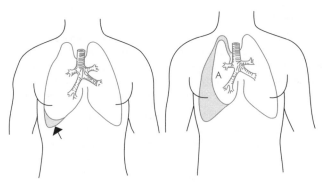

Figure 11.3 Pleural effusion. This starts as a small collection of fluid (arrow) between the lung and chest wall. If it increases it may gradually fill the pleural space on the side of the chest, compressing the lung (A).

a thin needle through the chest wall into the fluid and then suck it off with a needle and syringe. This is done under a local anaesthetic and is quite quick. As the fluid is being removed, the changing position of the lung may cause some discomfort and coughing. If the procedure becomes uncomfortable, tell the doctor as this is often an indication to stop because nearly all the fluid has been removed. Once the fluid has been removed a drug is usually inserted through the needle in the chest to try to prevent the fluid recurring. The fluid develops between the thick outer lining of the lung (parietal pleura) and the thin inner lining covering the lung (visceral pleura). The aim is to get these two parts of the lining of the lung to 'stick' together and thus prevent the fluid building up. Agents used include tetracycline (an antibiotic), 5-fluorouracil (5-FU: a chemotherapy drug), and talc. A chest X-ray will be taken after the procedure (called a pleurocentesis) to check that the fluid has gone and that no air has been allowed to leak into the pleural space (causing a pneumothorax).

If the fluid keeps coming back despite pleurocentesis, a minor operation may be done (under local anaesthetic) to pass a thin tube into the pleural fluid. This is left in place and is connected to a sealed water bottle (page 61). If necessary this may be connected to a pump that sucks out as much fluid as possible. When the pleural space is as 'dry' as possible, a drug may be injected through the tube to produce inflammation of the surfaces of the pleura in an attempt to produce scar tissue that will seal off the pleural space (pleurodesis). It this succeeds it will prevent the formation of a new effusion. Although the chest tube and drug both cause discomfort and require the patient to came into hospital for a day or two, the chances of success are about 50:50 so it is well worth trying if a pleural effusion keeps coming back. The type of drug injected through the tube varies, and some may cause a temporary burning discomfort or a fever, which can be helped by anti-inflammatory pain-killers such as aspirin.

Pleurocentesis

Sometimes pleurocentesis is performed under a general anaesthetic, the advantage being that it is easier for the surgeon to ensure all the fluid has been removed. Alternatively a new system has been developed that allows the fluid to be drained off intermittently and is introduced under local anaesthetic. This technique uses an indwelling pleural catheter that stays there permanently.

These silicone catheters are generally inserted using image guidance in the X-ray department and are tunnelled into the pleural space. The catheter has a one-way valve that prevents air from entering the chest cavity and fluid from coming out when not being drained. Once the catheter is placed and a chest X-ray has ruled out a pneumothorax, the patient can go home and manage the effusion as an outpatient. Two to three times per week, or as necessary, the patient or relative will need to drain the catheter using the appropriate supplies. Usually only 500–1,000 ml of fluid is removed at any one time, and fluid amounts usually decrease over time. Patients feel a sense of control with this catheter because it lets them be at home and not continuously connected to a drainage system for their remaining survival time. Neither do they have to have emergency unscheduled admissions to hospital to have the fluid drained off.

Pericardial effusion

What is it?

The heart is surrounded by a sac—the pericardium—which may fill with fluid, much as pleural fluid can fill the space between the chest wall and lungs (page 94). Because this sac is not very flexible, the fluid quickly fills it and starts to exert pressure on the beating heart. If the amount of fluid continues to increase it eventually affects the heart's pumping action, so that it starts to fail.

Because of the pressure the heart is not able to fill with blood properly and the back pressure causes fluid to build up in the lungs, and eventually in the body tissues. This results in increasing shortness of breath and swelling of the ankles. The blood pressure often falls and this causes the patient to feel dizzy, especially on suddenly standing up. These symptoms can be caused by many other things, changes in heart rhythm for instance, but if fluid is shown to be building up around the heart it often needs to be removed. The diagnosis of a pericardial effusion is made on clinical examination by a doctor and is confirmed by ultrasound examination of the heart. The usual cause of pericardial effusion in lung cancer is direct invasion of the cancer into the pericardium around the heart.

How can it be dealt with?

If a significant amount of fluid is found to be affecting the heart's action, the effusion must be drained. After an injection of local anaesthetic, a thin needle is passed between the ribs and carefully pushed forwards using an ultrasound machine called an echocardiogram to direct the needle until it is in the fluid around the heart, which is then sucked out. Provided that treatment can be given to control the tumour that is causing the build-up of fluid, this may be all that is necessary.

However, if fluid keeps building up it may become necessary to do a small operation to remove a portion (called a window) of the front of the pericardial sac. This allows the fluid to drain into the chest, where it is less of a problem. It is also possible to inject a drug into the pericardial sac in an attempt to try to stop the fluid coming back.

Hormone production by lung cancers

Any malignant tumour can produce hormones (chemical messengers that control the body's glands and some of its functions) but lung tumours, particularly small cell lung cancers, do so more often than any other type of cancer. Normally the amounts of various hormones in the body are very carefully regulated by a variety of delicate checks and balances. However, when a tumour produces a hormone it ignores these checks and balances and excessive amounts of the hormone are secreted into the bloodstream. The vast excess of the hormone causes abnormal changes in the body, the nature of which depend on the type of hormone being produced. Some of the more common problems are outlined below.

Corticosteroid (cortisol) excess

What is it?

Some lung tumours may secrete a hormone called ACTH (adrenocorticotrophic hormone), whose normal job is to stimulate the adrenal glands to produce steroid hormones. These will have a number of effects, which include:

- increased weight;
- deposition of fat over the face and trunk but not the limbs—this produces a round face (sometimes called a moon-face) and a fat pad over the shoulders;
- muscle weakness, which may become severe, affecting the large proximal muscles in the legs and arms; typical symptoms are difficulty in getting up out of the chair, climbing stairs, or combing hair;
- changes in the balance of salts (especially potassium in the blood) and a raised blood pressure.

How can it be dealt with?

The best way to treat this condition is to deal with the underlying cause—the tumour. If surgery, radiotherapy, or chemotherapy can shrink or get rid of the cancer, this relieves the symptoms. Drugs that block the production of the steroid hormones in the adrenal gland can be tried but control of the cancer is the only sure way to prevent the symptoms.

Excess antidiuretic hormone (ADH)

What is it?

This hormone is normally concerned with controlling how much water the kidneys retain in the body; it is frequently produced in small-cell lung cancer (page 6). Symptoms of excess production (known as the syndrome of inappropriate antidiuretic hormone or SIADH) include:

- loss of appetite;
- nausea and vomiting;
- lethargy;
- abnormal levels of salts in the blood (low sodium).

How can it be dealt with?

Treatment is preferably that of the underlying tumour that is overproducing the hormone (ADH). Because it is most commonly associated with small-cell cancers, this may be possible with chemotherapy, even when the tumour is widespread. Whilst treatment is being started, simple restriction of fluid intake, less than 1 litre per day, or the use of an antibiotic that interferes with the salt/water balance (demeclocycline), can improve the symptoms. It is very important to maintain the strict fluid intake because excess fluids can make the patient very unwell and can even lead to fits caused by the brain becoming waterlogged.

Excess calcium in blood (hypercalcaemia)

What is it?

This is particularly common in squamous lung cancer (page 7) and may be due to the overproduction of a hormone similar to parathyroid hormone by the tumour—this hormone controls the balance of calcium in the blood and the bones. Less commonly it may arise because there is extensive tumour in bone that releases calcium. The symptoms are:

- loss of appetite;
- nausea;
- excessive thirst and excessive urine production;
- constipation;
- bone pain;
- drowsiness that can lead to near-coma.

How can it be dealt with?

Treatment is, as in similar situations, that of the underlying tumour. While treatment is being started the symptoms may be helped by a high fluid intake (by a drip into a vein if necessary) and use of new drugs that control calcium called biphosphonates such as pamidronate or zoledronic acid.

Other hormone syndromes

Many other different types of hormones may be produced by lung cancers but this is relatively uncommon.

Spread of lung cancer to the bones

Spread of lung cancer to the bones is unfortunately fairly common late in the course of the disease. Pain is the most frequent symptom. Because the bones are weakened by the tumour, breaks or fractures can occur after even minor injury.

Local treatment to the bone

Treatment is usually with radiotherapy to the painful bone or fracture, although some fractures in bones in the arms or legs will need special support. This usually means a small operation to put a steel pin down the centre of the bone to give it stability and fix the fracture. Radiotherapy is usually very good at relieving bone pain in 80% of cases but pain-killing medicines will likely be necessary before treatment works. The average time for radiotherapy to reduce the pain is about 3 weeks. Anti-inflammatory drugs such as ibuprofen seem to be particularly good at reducing bone pain and can be added to other pain-killing drugs (see below). Figure 11.4 shows the World Health Organization (WHO) approach or ladder for pain-killers. The weaker medications are given in maximum dose before the stronger medications such as morphine are used.

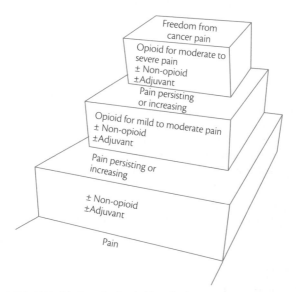

Figure 11.4 World Health Organization ladder of pain control.

Source: reproduced with permission from WHO, http://www.who.int/cancer/palliative/painladder/en/

This reduces the risk of the inevitable side-effects, particularly constipation that comes with the stronger medications. Drugs such as ibuprofen are used with the pain-killers to increase the effectiveness.

General treatments

Biphosphonates are drugs that are commonly used to treat osteoporosis (bone thinning). Newer-generation bisphosphonates have now been shown to reduce the complications that can arise when cancer spreads to bones. These are called 'skeletal-related events' (SREs) and include pain, hypercalcaemia (raised calcium in the blood), bone fractures, and spinal cord and nerve compression. These are all very unpleasant problems and it is not surprising that preventing them can lead to improvements in the quality of life of patients with metastatic bone disease who are likely to have a prolonged clinical course. Indeed there is a suggestion that they may be just as effective as radiotherapy, which remains the standard treatment for pain relief when cancer has spread to the bone.

Swelling of the bones at the fingertip together with curvature of the nails (clubbing) is quite common in lung cancer. In some patients this may progress to painful swellings at various joints, called hypertrophic pulmonary osteoarthropathy. The only way of improving these is successful treatment of the cancer itself, which suggests that it is caused by something produced by the cancer. If it is not possible to shrink the cancer, anti-inflammatory pain-killers and sometimes steroids can be used to reduce the discomfort.

Spread of lung cancer to the brain or nerves
Brain

The idea of a tumour affecting the brain is terrifying because it seems to attack the centre of our very being. Unfortunately, lung cancers can spread to the brain and cause all sorts of different symptoms. Nevertheless, these can often be controlled and only occur in a minority of patients. Spread to the brain is most often seen in small-cell lung cancer and is more common when patients have responded well to their treatment and have lived for longer periods. This allows the tumour the chance to grow in the brain, the one place where the drugs may not have reached (page 79). For this reason, some patients with small-cell lung cancer receive brain radiotherapy after initial chemotherapy.

If a tumour does affect the brain, it can produce many different symptoms according to which part of the brain is affected. The common symptoms are:

- severe headache—usually worse on waking and made worse by straining or coughing;
- nausea and vomiting;
- weakness of part of the body;
- change of feeling in part of the body;
- disturbance in balance;

* disturbance of vision;
* change in mood;
* fits, as in epilepsy.

If spread of lung cancer to the brain is found, usually by computed tomography (CT) scan or magnetic resonance imaging (MRI) (page 53), radiotherapy either to the whole brain or targeted to the cancer deposits is generally given; surgery is rarely indicated. Steroid treatment with the drug dexamethasone is often used first, to reduce any inflammation and swelling (oedema) around the tumour. Because the brain is enclosed in the bony skull, any swelling rapidly causes pressure on the brain, which causes headache and other symptoms. Dexamethasone usually relieves this promptly and reduces the symptoms. If a fit has occurred, anti-epileptic drugs—generally sodium valproate, carbamezepine or phenytoin—will be given to try prevent any more occurring.

Radiotherapy can shrink the tumour. Unfortunately chemotherapy does not cross the blood–brain barrier and thus is rarely prescribed. Although the response to treatment is often dramatic, it is unfortunately often temporary, although it can be useful in reducing symptoms.

Spinal cord

Occasionally a lung tumour may spread to affect the spinal cord rather than the brain. This will cause:

* weakness, usually in both legs;
* loss or change in sensation in the lower part of the body—the upper level of this loss of feeling depends on the site of the tumour;
* disturbed bowel and bladder function so that normal control is lost.

Anyone with these symptoms should see a doctor *immediately*, as it is of the utmost urgency that treatment is started early. Symptoms which are allowed to progress may become permanent. If an early operation (to relieve the pressure on the spine) or radiotherapy is given then there is a chance of at least some recovery. Dexamethasone should be started as soon as the diagnosis is suspected to reduce any swelling and oedema. Patients with the symptoms or signs of pressure on the spinal cord should be referred to a neurosurgeon or radiotherapist immediately and will undergo an urgent MRI scan of the whole spine. Undue delay risks permanent loss of power in the legs with loss of bowel and bladder function (paraplegia).

Nerves

Pressure from the tumour on a nerve will damage it and often stop it working normally. The most common places for this to happen in patients with lung cancer are in the centre of the chest and in the neck. The nerve to the left side of the larynx loops down into the chest near the heart and a tumour involving lymph glands in the left side of the chest may press on it, causing marked hoarseness. This is because the left-hand vocal cord no longer receives messages from the brain and cannot move. An injection of teflon directly into the vocal cord can be used to try to improve the hoarseness but there is rarely any treatment that will cause the nerve to start working normally after it has been damaged.

Similarly, when tumours develop in the top part of the lung (superior sulcus tumours), they may affect a special nerve that supplies the eye. This will cause drooping of the eyelid on that side, a contracted pupil, and a slightly depressed eyeball—a condition known as Horner's syndrome. Although it is not dangerous in itself it is troublesome, as it responds poorly to treatment even if the tumour shrinks. Tumours in this area can also involve the complex sheath of nerves supplying the arm (the brachial plexus) and pressure can lead to pain, weakness, and altered sensation.

Generalized effects on the nerves and brain

A few patients develop symptoms, often before there is any sign of lung cancer, that cannot be explained by the presence of cancer pressing on, or directly infiltrating, the nervous system. These so-called paraneoplastic phenomena and can improve when the cancer is treated. It is believed that such symptoms are caused by chemicals that damage the nervous system—the chemicals being produced by the tumour itself.

The common symptoms are:

- weakness of muscles;
- loss of balance;
- change in sensation or feeling;
- muscle weakness and pain with wasting of the muscles.

These sorts of symptoms are very general in their nature and are very common, so that it is important to remember that only very rarely are they due to a developing lung cancer.

Skin rashes

Occasionally a cancer that starts in the lung may grow under or in the skin. Such growths appear as a nodular area in the skin. This raised area is often purplish, can form an ulcer and bleed, and may be uncomfortable. Radiotherapy or chemotherapy may be able to shrink it down and pain-killers may be needed. There is no danger of severe bleeding.

Some patients with cancer may develop skin changes that are not directly caused by invasion of the skin by the tumour. It seems likely that they are caused by chemicals produced by the tumour itself, as they tend to improve when the cancer is removed. There are a wide variety of these skin rashes, although they are all rather uncommon. Some patients develop extensive dark pigmented areas, especially under the arms, whilst others have scaly or blistered areas. Occasionally these rashes may be associated with muscle pain and weakness (a condition called dermato-myositis). Most patients with lung cancer do not have one of these syndromes, and certainly anyone with a rash is very unlikely to turn out to have cancer.

Treatment of the underlying cancer is the surest way to improve the rash, although steroids can be helpful, particularly if muscle pains and weakness are present.

Cough

A cough is the most common symptom caused by lung cancer and can be continuous and very trying. Any treatment that can get rid of the cancer itself is the best way of dealing with it. However, if this is not possible it can usually be helped with various cough suppressants. These, in increasing strength, include:

- codeine linctus;
- pholcodine linctus;
- methadone linctus;
- oral morphine sulphate.

Other types of cough medicine may be used:

- expectorants that stimulate the cough to try to help clear the lung secretion;
- mucolytics, designed to reduce the thickness of any phlegm so that it is brought up more easily.

For most patients a cough suppressant is all that is required, although a mucolytic may be helpful in some patients.

Pain

Many people think of cancer as a fatal disease in which pain is always a problem. In fact, about a half of patients with advancing cancer do not have significant pain but, for those who do, expert care can ensure that it is kept under control.

Pain in lung cancer is most commonly due to invasion into the chest wall or sensitive structures in the chest, or due to spread of tumour into the bones. If radiotherapy or chemotherapy can be used to shrink the tumour, this is obviously the best way of dealing with the problem. If this is not possible, appropriate use of pain-killers and other drugs can control most of the pain and discomfort.

Pain often varies in severity during the day and is usually worse at night. This may be partly due to the use of drugs that ease pain for a while and then allow it to return, although it is also largely related to mood. Pain is not just a simple physical sensation, it is very greatly influenced and made worse by depression, anxiety, and all sorts of stress. Chronic pain can take over one's life, if it:

- seems to be without a foreseeable end;
- tends to get worse rather than better;
- serves no purpose;
- takes up all your attention and can make life not seem worth living.

This type of pain needs expert treatment and in most cases can be controlled, making life worthwhile again.

Using pain-killers

The essence of controlling pain is to give an effective dose of a pain-killer often enough to keep the pain at bay at all times. This sounds obvious, but all too often patients, doctors, and nurses are reluctant to use frequent doses of strong pain-killers. It is never helpful to use pain-killers only when the pain is bad; this tends to lead to gradually increasing doses to control the worsening pain.

For instance, if after taking a pain-killer patients are pain-free for 4.5–5 hours, they will need to take the next dose after 4 hours, so that the drug has been fully absorbed before the pain returns. It is best to give pain-killers by mouth and injections can be avoided in nearly all patients. It is important to remember that, when powerful pain-killers are being used to control pain, addiction is not a real problem. Regular doses of drugs such as morphine may be taken quite safely. Interestingly if the pain goes then the morphine can be stopped quite quickly without withdrawal symptoms.

Unless pain is very severe, it is best to start with simple pain-killers and to increase the strength gradually until the pain is controlled. Some of the drugs used are shown below but many others are also available. Figure 11.4 shows the recommendations used internationally as advised by the WHO and known as the WHO ladder for pain-killers. The weaker medications are given in maximum dose before stronger medications such as morphine are used. This reduces the risk of the inevitable side-effects, particularly constipation that comes with the stronger medications.

Mild pain

This is usually well treated by aspirin or paracetamol. One or two tablets should be taken every 4 hours.

Moderate pain

If aspirin or paracetamol are insufficient, weak narcotic drugs can be used. These often contain a combination of drugs, usually including codeine. The commonly prescribed drugs are:

- co-codamol (paracetamol and dihydrocodeine);
- codeine phosphate.

The usual dose is one or two tablets every 4 hours. There are many other similar drugs; all require a doctor's prescription.

Severe pain

Stronger narcotic drugs are usually needed and can be given safely and regularly and are always worth trying. The dose can often be reduced once the pain is under control. Some may cause sleepiness, and loss of concentration is common at first, although this gradually improves as the body gets used to the pain-killer. Fortunately, the pain continues to be controlled by the same dose, and increasing doses are not normally needed once the right dose has been found. Available drugs include:

- slow-release morphine with the advantage that it only need be taken twice a day;
- morphine sulphate solution;
- oxycodone, a morphine-like drug, possibly less constipating than morphine;
- tramadol: is a centrally acting analgesic;
- buprenorphine (Temgesic®): a moderately strong narcotic that can be sucked under the tongue;
- fentanyl patches.

At first these drugs are given in quick-acting preparations. The right dose for you can then be found and then converted to longer-acting preparations given twice a day. This stops the sleep disturbance that is common with swift-acting drugs. All pain-killers are best given by mouth on a regular basis. Stronger pain-killers all constipate and it is normal to routinely prescribe a strong laxative with them.

Pain is much worse if depression or stress is a problem and the use of appropriate drugs to deal with depression and anxiety are very helpful in getting pain under control. When bone or nerve pain is a problem, anti-inflammatory drugs can be very helpful in addition to the ordinary pain-killers.

Perhaps one of the most important ways doctors, nurses, and families can help patients with pain is to take the time to listen to them. Isolation and depression make it much more difficult to control the pain and half an hour spent listening to and talking with a patient may mean that the efficacy of a drug is greatly increased.

Other ways of stopping pain

If drugs are not entirely effective, other methods can be tried.

Nerve blocks

Because pain sensations are carried by nerves, anything that damages nerves and blocks their ability to carry messages can reduce the feeling of pain. Injections of local anaesthetic or substances designed to damage nerves can be given. They can be helpful in particular cases, although in some instances there is a risk that they may damage the function of the part of the body supplied by the nerve that has been injected. Because of this it is important to discuss with the doctor the advantages and disadvantages of such treatment. Nerve blocks are usually only available in special pain clinics.

Transcutaneous nerve stimulation (TNS)
Electrical stimulation of skin near a painful area may reduce the pain itself. Unfortunately the effect is usually quite temporary.

Hypnosis
This can be used together with other methods of pain control but is usually only of temporary benefit. Its main value may be that the doctor spends half an hour with the patient.

Acupuncture
This seems to give temporary relief of pain to some patients, but has so far been little used in cancer patients.

Loss of appetite and weight

This is very common when a patient has a growing tumour and may be due to several factors:

- The tumour may be altering the body's metabolism and burning up excessive amounts of energy.

- The tumour and its treatment may be causing nausea and vomiting, diarrhoea, or failure to absorb food that is eaten.

- Tumours sometimes cause patients to feel revolted by the sight or smell of food—they just do not feel like eating.

- Anxiety.

Prolonged loss of appetite, called anorexia, leads to wasting, which is known as cachexia. This is difficult to treat as the more weight patients lose, the less they feel like eating. Family and friends are concerned and often press the patient to eat, which usually only makes things worse.

It is best for patients to try to eat small regular meals of anything that they fancy. Foods with a strong smell should be avoided and things that look attractive should be chosen. A drink of alcohol or a tonic before eating may help but the use of steroids (prednisolone or dexamethasone) is usually the surest way of improving appetite. Prednisolone, in addition to improving appetite, usually gives a general feeling of well-being. Alternatively, megestrol acetate (a hormone used to treat breast cancer) may be used to stimulate appetite—it has the advantage of not causing the side-effects of steroids.

Food supplements can be helpful and supply calories and protein. The main problem is that it is often difficult to find a flavour that is palatable. It is often worth trying a sample of different flavours of various food supplements to see if there is one that is more palatable than the others.

The important features of pain control are as follows:

- Pain is not only physical; treatment of depression and anxiety or even just the opportunity to discuss their illness and feelings is a great help to most patients.
- Severe pain can nearly always be, at least partially, controlled.
- A sufficiently strong drug must be used regularly so that unacceptable pain does not return between doses.
- Narcotic drugs do not cause addiction if used to control pain.
- Other methods are available if drugs do not work.

Part 3
Dealing with lung cancer

12

Getting the best treatment

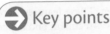 Key points

- There is a national priority to improve cancer treatments and outcomes.
- Your care will be coordinated by a specialist multidisciplinary team.
- Your GP can refer urgently to the specialist team if cancer is suspected.
- National targets exist to ensure that you are promptly treated.
- National guidelines exist to ensure that patients throughout the country have access to best care.

NHS Cancer Plan 2000

There was general recognition in the 1990s that the National Health Service (NHS) was underfunded, often with long waits for treatment and not enough specialist staff. There was also clear evidence of worse survival for all types of cancer in the UK compared to the rest of Europe. As a result in 2000 an NHS cancer plan was launched. This was based on the government's public health strategy, *Our Healthier Nation*, which set a target to reduce cancer deaths in the under 65s by a fifth by the year 2010. Part of the approach included establishing a set of national cancer standards that are monitored by a process called peer review. These tell health professionals what standards of care are expected, and in particular how services should be organized to make sure that patients get best care. Some of these plans arose from a survey in Scotland.

Scotland leads international tables in both incidence and mortality from lung cancer. This has been due, historically, to a high prevalence of smoking, perhaps coupled with poor diet and some industrial exposures. Survival from lung cancer is poor in Scotland when compared internationally, and factors that seemed to account for this included:

- delays in presentation to doctors;
- other medical problems which mean that aggressive treatment cannot be given;

- delays in investigation;
- delays in treatment;
- lack of specialty working;
- lack of access to specialist advice and treatment;
- undertreatment or therapeutic nihilism, i.e. the doctors do not believe that treatment helps;
- more accurate cancer registration data compared to the rest of Europe, in other words in the UK our systems are better at counting the true numbers of cancer cases.

The Scottish study showed that, when patients were seen by a chest physician, oncologist, or thoracic surgeon, patients did better. These features were an independent predictor of access to potentially curative treatment and hence better survival. In other words if you see the correct specialist you are more likely to get the best treatment.

Clearly it is important to ensure that patients receive the best treatment using current knowledge for their stage of disease. This is about quality of care and seeing a specialist with a special interest in lung cancer who works within a specialist multidisciplinary team. The national cancer standards have resulted in the establishment of specialist teams in most hospitals in England. If that team is not present in your hospital you should expect to be referred to such a team in a nearby hospital. The lung cancer team should include medical and nursing staff with specialized knowledge of diagnosis and treatment, both curative and palliative, of lung cancer. They will assess you and almost certainly introduce you to a specialist nurse who will be your 'key worker', namely a point of contact with the hospital team throughout your illness.

The multidisciplinary team

The composition of the multidisciplinary lung cancer team should include the following:

- Lead clinician—normally a respiratory physician—who should take managerial responsibility for the service as a whole.
- Respiratory (chest) physician with a special interest in lung cancer.
- Radiologist (interprets X-rays) with chest expertise. The radiologist will normally ensure that when a chest X-ray is taken for another reason, say at the request of your GP, and it shows a possible lung cancer it is automatically flagged up and referred to the lung cancer team.
- Pathologist ± cytologist who interprets biopsy samples.
- Nurse specialist: nominated individual with specialized knowledge of lung disease and cancer who should be available to provide patient support and advocacy, to facilitate communication and the flow of information, and to liaise with other services.

- Oncologist, preferably with a special interest in lung cancer: either a clinical oncologist, otherwise known as radiotherapist, who can offer both radio- and chemotherapy, or a medical oncologist who specializes in cancer drug therapies who must work closely with a clinical oncologist from the centre to which patients are referred for radiotherapy.

- Palliative care specialist: because of the nature of the disease, close links with the palliative care team are essential.

- Thoracic surgeon, who may be a core member of one or more teams and should be involved in developing local clinical policy and audit. She/he may not attend all meetings but should be readily available to liaise with the lung cancer team when required and to ensure that patients who may benefit from surgery are assessed promptly. The surgeon will coordinate local surgical policy.

The palliative care team should also be multiprofessional and should, as a minimum, include the following members:

- palliative care physician;
- palliative care nurse specialists.

In addition, the team should include, or have close links with, the following:

- psychologist/psychiatrist;
- social worker;
- chaplain/pastoral care worker;
- bereavement care worker;
- primary healthcare team.

The multidisciplinary care team's role includes both direct care for patients and families with lung cancer but also the provision of advice, support, and education for other health professionals who are involved in patient care. The team will usually meet weekly and must discuss any new case diagnosed with lung cancer. They are also likely to discuss situations when patients are having problems, such that a different treatment approach is needed. When the team have met, their advice and opinions will be discussed with you. If you do not want what the team has suggested, that is absolutely fine—your choice remains extremely important. For example, many patients are clear that they do not want chemotherapy treatment.

National cancer standards

National guidance on the organization and development of services and treatments are determined nationally. They are contained in *Guidance on Commissioning Services* published by the National Institute for Health and Clinical Excellence and called 'Improving Outcomes in Lung Cancer'. This will be updated every few years, and is available online for both patients and healthcare professionals to reference.

The document reviews the available evidence for all stages of the disease and bases its advice on that information. Each topic area includes five sections which summarize:

* the recommendations;
* potential benefits of implementing them to patients and the NHS;
* the strength of the supporting evidence;
* how implementation may be measured;
* the resource implications to the NHS of implementing the recommendations.

The topic areas are:

* Prevention.
* Access, diagnosis, and staging.
* Multiprofessional teams.
* Communication, information, and support.
* Radical treatment for non-small cell lung cancer (NSCLC).
* Radical treatment for small cell lung cancer (SCLC).
* Palliative interventions and care.

One major key is patient-centred care with a priority given to communication and support for patients, which previously has been one of the major complaints that patients had against the NHS. For example, some of the key recommendations include that patients should have 'quick access to appropriate team members throughout the course of their illness'. Others are that 'palliative care should be an integral part of patient management from the outset' and that 'Palliative care should be the responsibility of a multiprofessional team which has close links with the lung cancer team, sharing at least one member in common.'

Getting referred to the multidisiciplinary team: the 2-week wait rule

As part of the cancer plan, time scales for both investigation and treatment were made.

For patients with suspected cancer the GP can refer under a system called the '2-week wait rule'. This means that referral to the specialist lung team is urgent and either further tests must be done or the patient seen within 2 weeks of the doctor faxing the referral, often electronically, to the specialist lung cancer team. Most hospitals have guidance for the use of the 2-week rule but common criteria that qualify for referral include:

* chest X-ray suggestive/suspicious of lung cancer (including pleural effusion and slowly resolving infection);

◆ persistent haemoptysis (coughing up blood) in smokers/ex-smokers over 40 years of age;

◆ signs of superior vena caval obstruction (swelling of face/neck with fixed elevation of jugular venous pressure);

◆ stridor (noisy breathing due to narrowing of the airway) (GPs are advised to consider emergency referral).

Once a referral has been made there are additional rules: first that a diagnosis must be made within 31 days of referral and second that treatment must start within 62 days of referral, or within 31 days from the date of the diagnosis being made.

Hospitals are set targets for the number of cases referred that must be met for these goals and they are currently that:

◆ 100% of cases must meet the 2-week rule;

◆ 98% of cases must meet the 31-day rule;

◆ 95% of cases must meet the 62-day rule.

Other methods of referral

The vast majority of patients (nine out of ten) referred by their GP under the 2-week rule with a suspicion of cancer turn out not to have cancer at all. Likewise less than half of all cancers are diagnosed through the 2-week rule pathway. For example, lung cancer may be diagnosed during a patient's emergency admission to hospital with a chest infection or incidentally during investigation of another problem. If that happens to you, you should expect to be referred to the multidisciplinary team and the national standard of treatment within 31 days of diagnosis still holds.

National Institute for Health and Clinical Excellence (NICE)

NICE was established as part of the NHS reforms in 2000. NICE is an independent organization responsible for providing national guidance on the promotion of good health and the prevention and treatment of ill health. NICE currently advises about current best practice for treatment and investigation of all diseases. Two particular areas of NICE's work impact on lung cancer:

◆ *Health technologies:* guidance on the use of new and existing medicines, treatments, and procedures within the NHS. Here the objective is to determine those treatments that should be made available within the limited resources of the NHS and also those that should not.

◆ *Clinical practice:* guidance on the appropriate treatment and care of people with specific diseases and conditions within the NHS. There are specific guidelines for lung cancer.

The NICE website (Appendix) provides a good source of relevant information.

Second opinions

If you are unsure whether either you or your family members are getting the best treatment, for what ever reason, you have the right to ask for a second opinion from another healthcare professional. Your GP can refer you for that advice.

13

Living with lung cancer

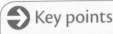 **Key points**

- It's best to talk openly about your cancer.

- A good diet and exercise seem to help deal with the illness and may prolong the length of life.

- Beware of dangerous claims for drugs and other approaches on the internet.

- More people are alive after successful treatment for cancer. Their needs are increasingly recognized and called survivorship.

For most people cancer is a dreaded disease and cancer of the lung is particularly feared. Treatment remains disappointing and because of the clear association with smoking there is often a lot of self-blame. Because of this, it is often a subject shrouded in secrecy and thus the opportunity for misinformation is huge. Nowadays, however, people are more open in talking about cancer than previous generations. If you have read the rest of this book you will have found that, unfortunately, very many patients with lung cancer do die of their tumour, but there are some who are cured and most others can now benefit from treatment. Better communication skills training has made doctors understand that most patients want to know what is happening to them, but also want to know all about their illness and treatment—even if the news is not good.

Uncertainty

For the majority, fear of the unknown and uncertainty is more frightening and much more difficult to cope with than the truth. Nowadays patients are told at the same time as the family, removing a potentially very destructive situation in which no-one can discuss what is happening for fear of causing distress, even though everyone, including the patient, deep down knows what is happening.

In most situations you and your family should expect a straightforward explanation of the disease and its treatment. You should expect any questions to be answered with honesty, but tempered with sensitivity. If there is good information as well as bad, this should be given as soon as possible in a realistic manner.

It is very important for patients to develop a good relationship with their doctors and nurses and, as mentioned before, this book is intended only as a back-up. It is hoped that it will help to develop open discussion by prompting questions as well as providing practical information and sources of help.

Once the diagnosis of lung cancer is out in the open it is then possible to discuss how it is going to be handled. Discussions about tests, treatment, and the outlook will hopefully proceed at a pace that the patient can handle comfortably: if patients are allowed to lead the discussion this is ensured. Family, doctors, and nurses need to learn to *listen* to patients, their frustrations, worries, and questions. Anyone with cancer is under severe stress from the first time they realize what the trouble may be, and they will continue to have emotional ups and downs during the course of the disease. Don't worry if you need to have the same thing repeated lots of times—we can only absorb a limited amount of information and often it needs to be repeated so that we can fully understand.

Finding out about your illness

Very often, discovering a symptom (such as coughing up blood) that suggests cancer to the individual can be even more shocking than actually finding out that it *is* cancer.

Once the diagnosis is confirmed you will be allocated a specialist nurse whom you can contact as you need, and who will support you through both the diagnostic tests needed and also any treatment and follow-up. Your nurse will have specific knowledge about your condition. In addition you will be given written information about the tests to be performed, which you can read at your own pace. The internet is a wonderful additional resource but can also be a trap for the unwary. Anyone can put any information of any type, however outrageously inaccurate, onto the internet. It is safer to stick to the recommended major websites run by the major cancer charities.

One of the biggest crises for patients with cancer is loss of control of their own life. Suddenly struck with cancer, they are taken over by the hospital and seemingly have no power over their destiny. Inclusion of those patients who wish it into the whole process of diagnosis and treatment goes a good way to reducing their feeling of helplessness. Patients who want to ask questions may find it helpful to write them down; it is only too easy to forget what they were, during the stress of seeing the doctor.

Support organizations, such as the Roy Castle Lung Cancer Foundation or Macmillan, can answer many questions for patients and their families. They can also supply much relevant information, including details on support groups, etc. These and other organizations are listed in the Appendix with appropriate addresses, websites, and telephone numbers.

Living with cancer

The 'war on cancer'

One of the commonest questions we get asked as cancer specialists is 'What can I do to help myself?' We usually think of having cancer as a battle. Indeed the 'war against cancer' was launched by President Nixon in the USA in 1971. He said 'I will launch an intensive campaign to find a cure for cancer, and I will ask later for whatever additional funds can effectively be used. The time has come in America when the same kind of concentrated effort that split the atom and took man to the moon should be turned toward conquering this dread disease. Let us make a total national commitment to achieve this goal.' There has been progress—survival rates are slowly improving, and basic research has developed hugely—but the war has not been won in that the number of people getting cancer continues to rise. Currently one in three people can expect to get cancer at some stage in their lives and this will rise to one in two by 2020.

So if the 'war' on cancer has been lost what can we expect in the future? We need to learn to live with cancer just as we do with other serious illnesses. For example, diabetes currently cannot be cured but, with modification of diet and additional drugs such as insulin when necessary, the symptoms and organ-damaging and thus fatal effects of the illness can be controlled. It is a chronic illness, like HIV AIDS (human immunodeficiency virus; acquired immunodeficiency syndrome). When AIDS was discovered in the early 1980s it was feared, just like cancer, as a progressive and rapidly fatal illness. Now advances in antiviral treatment mean that the disease can be effectively controlled for years. The same situation is likely to develop in cancer treatments. Although new biological or targeted agents are exciting steps forward, they are more likely to control the disease rather than cure. Thus cancer will, for many, become a chronic disease just like diabetes, and controlled rather than cured by treatment.

One important emphasis is well-being, not illness. Thus the question 'What can I do for myself to cope with and live with cancer?' is at least as important as specific anticancer treatments.

Exercise

It's hard not to hear about the benefits of exercise these days. There is very good evidence that the risk of colon cancer developing can be reduced by increased physical activity. The data for lung cancer are not so clear-cut. However, it is likely that being physically active not only helps prevent lung cancer in the first place, but may improve survival and quality of life for those already diagnosed. One study found that physical activity was linked with a lower risk of developing lung cancer. The benefit extended to everyone; men and women, as well as those who were smokers, former smokers, or had never touched a cigarette. The activities looked at by researchers did not require hours per day or health club membership. Even gardening twice a week was associated with a reduced risk.

That patients are increasingly seeking guidance on physical activity was shown in an analysis of 300 lung cancer patients' requests. Sixty per cent wanted some instruction, and 77% of those wanted instruction from a specialist in physical education at a cancer centre. Most want instruction before treatment. This shows the need for advice in addition to treatment, not least showing that we need to understand better which type of exercise can benefit lung cancer patients.

Physical activity appears to improve quality of life for those with cancer in general. It also has been found to decrease cancer-related fatigue and tiredness, one of the most distressing and common symptoms for many with cancer. Even those who have undergone surgery to remove lung cancer can tolerate and benefit from exercise regimens starting just a month after surgery.

Fatigue is one of the most frequent side-effects of chemotherapy. Participants in exercise programmes tend to experience physical fatigue in the experimental project period that was considered positive compared to the negative chemotherapy-induced fatigue. Patients seem to learn how to handle the intense fatigue by using exercise to stop the feelings of physical weakness. Patients tell us that they feel more energetic and that exercise increases their physical well-being.

Diet and vitamins

The relationship between diet and lung cancer has been examined in several epidemiological studies. Among persons with a high intake of fruit and vegetables, retrospective studies have shown halving the risk of lung cancer compared to persons with a low intake of fruit and vegetables. The results of prospective studies have been less conclusive, with a variation of 0–30% reduction in the risk of developing lung cancer. In the positive studies, the risk reduction was not dependent on smoking habits. There are currently no good published studies of the effects on cancer outcomes when diet is modified after cancer has been diagnosed. However, many patients find that modifying their lifestyles is positive in terms of their general well-being. This is worthwhile in itself even if it does not make people live longer.

For patients on active treatment it is important that they do not lose any weight. Patients with reduced appetite should try eating small and frequent meals, and what they fancy. Many treatments cause altered tastes, and sticking to a rigid diet can be difficult. After ending treatment a normal diet is recommended with lots of fruits and vegetables.

Many cancer sufferers take vitamin supplements at some stage in their illness. Whether vitamin supplements improve either quality or quantity of life is not known. One questionnaire has suggested that among the 63% who took dietary supplements, there was an increased chance of survival as well as a better score in life quality compared to the others. However, these results should be viewed with considerable caution since it was not a clinical study, and therefore bias may have occurred. Results from several prospective studies of specific vitamin supplements' effect on lung cancer are thus awaited.

Alternative treatments

The description 'alternative treatment' refers to treatments that go beyond the options usually offered by conventional health services and usually fall outwith the normal legal frameworks and licensing legislation which govern medicines. Examples include natural medicines and acupuncture. In our centre in Bristol at least 90% of patients have tried some form of alternative treatment at some point during their cancer diagnosis and treatment. The use of alternative treatment is not due to dissatisfaction with doctors. However, four out of ten users felt that they had been given little or hardly any hope from their doctors compared to two out of ten among the non-users. The implication is that cancer patients consider alternative treatment as a supplement rather than as an alternative to established treatments. Perhaps this is not surprising given the poor prognosis for many lung cancer patients. We all hope for full recovery and relief from the stark reality of the illness, but patients also seek feelings of hope, compassion, and spirituality that alternative approaches can provide. These needs are understandable to most practitioners in the established health care system, but they can be hard to satisfy. This is partly because of time pressures, but also because the doctor often has to bring bad news and carry out unpleasant treatments. You may be surprised but the majority of oncologists will support patients in their use of alternative treatment, although most will not encourage patients directly unless specifically asked.

The increased use of alternative treatments has made doctors consider changing negative preconceived attitudes, but also means that alternative therapists are now expected to do research to justify their claims for treatments. Not only must the studies show benefits to patients but also just like conventional remedies must be shown not to do harm. Only a few studies exist exploring lung cancer and alternative treatments.

Antioxidants

The use of antioxidants, e.g. vitamin C and Q_{10}, has been the subject of some research, but there remains disagreement when it comes to the possible benefits of these as either prevention or treatment.

Antioxidants used in large doses for cancer patients, either alone or as a supplement to chemo- and radiotherapy, have been tested in small clinical studies, though without conclusive results. Several oncologists are concerned about the use of antioxidants, since it is possible that they may counter the effects from various types of treatment. More specifically, there is a specific reason to warn against taking Echinacea, which can be found in several natural medicines and diet supplements. Simultaneous use of Echinacea and chemotherapy containing methotrexate might trigger an inflammation of the liver called hepatitis.

Acupuncture

Acupuncture plays an increasing part of smoking cessation. However, a Cochrane review which overviews all published materials found that acupuncture was no better than placebo or other interventions in regard to helping people stop smoking. However, there was some evidence that acupuncture might relieve pain, nausea and vomiting in connection with cancer treatment.

> Overall, the majority of cancer patients will seek alternative treatment at some point. It is important to tell your doctor what you are planning to do or take, in order to check that it is safe with your normal medication and cancer treatment.

Lung cancer and psychological reactions

Many studies have shown that patients have considerable stress and psychological effects with a diagnosis of cancer. Importantly cancer affects whole families and the stress and distress of the disease can often be worse for patient's partners who have to deal with the consequences of the illness. These reactions have been studied in detail in women with breast cancer. No study has specifically covered this area for patients with lung cancer. In animals increased stress can impact on progression of cancer, among other things through an effect on the immune system. Such a connection has never been shown in human cancer. In a large Danish study, the relationship between severe depression and the progression of breast cancer was examined, and it was found that patients with former or present depression did not have a higher risk of developing breast cancer. By contrast, breast cancer patients had a higher risk of getting a depression than others.

Some studies provide an image of lung cancer patients as human beings with reduced quality of life, increased mental stress and increased risk of depression. These tendencies are stronger with patients with a bad prognosis, among patients with physical symptoms of lung cancer (in particular shortness of breath and pain) and among those who are not being offered active treatment for their cancer. For those studies in which something was done, it was demonstrated that psychosocial intervention in the follow-up period after active treatment reduced physical symptoms, increased quality of life and reduced the risk of developing depression in the process of the lung cancer disease. These interventions have included spending time talking, home visits, providing written information about the possibilities for symptom relief, and regular contact with nurses or doctors. Since up to one-third of patients with cancer will develop a depressive illness during the course of their disease, these are potentially important findings. We need to understand better how to deal with and prevent the mental trauma that goes with a diagnosis of cancer.

Living life after cancer

How we live after treatment of cancer is called survivorship. As more people are cured of cancer they have to live with the after-effects of treatment and financial and psychological issues that arise. Most countries are developing survivorship programmes. The National Cancer Survivorship Initiative (NCSI) aims to provide better support to cancer survivors focusing on the following areas:

* assessment and care planning;
* managing active and progressive disease;
* late effects;
* children and young people;
* work and finance;
* self-management;
* research;
* information;
* workforce development and commissioning.

 Case study

John was diagnosed with advanced incurable lung cancer. His daughter Sharon did not want to believe he could not survive. She found a diet on a website from the USA which said that miracle cures were possible. The cost was high and she had no money. The website wanted $1,500 per month for the diet. A quick search revealed that the website owner was under conviction within the USA for fraud and stealing funds. We persuaded Sharon that she should save her money and take her father to the Penny Brohn centre, formerly the cancer help centre in Bristol. The family went for an introductory weekend and learned of various alternative approaches including diet and relaxation.

Beware of internet advertising. Ask if you are uncertain. Your cancer nurse is a good source of information.

14

Clinical trials

 Key points

- Trials are necessary to show that new approaches in medicine are safe and benefit patients.
- Clinical trials exist because progress in medicine is slow.
- Many of our current treatments are only in practice because patients took part in trials.
- Taking part in trials offers patients access to the most up-to-date care and treatments.

Before any new treatment can be offered to patients, whether it be a medicine, surgical treatment or device, it has to be tested to see not only whether is it effective, but also to check that it is safe. Such tests in patients are called clinical trials. The UK is proud of its record of more than doubling the number of cancer patients treated within clinical trials in just 3 years. It is not generally known but a greater proportion of cancer patients in the UK enter clinical trials than any other country in the world, including the USA. Trials exist because progress in medicine is not as quick as we would wish. If a new approach definitely cured all cancers with few side-effects it would need a large trial to be used, it would be obvious. Although trials are done of a number of approaches to treatment and investigation of cancer, the way new drugs are tested provides the best example of how trials are run.

Different types of trials

Trials have to answer different questions which depend on the knowledge that we already have about a treatment, and the type of intervention considered. Because of this, clinical trials are run in various ways.

Phase I trials

These are the first studies of a new drug in man. The drug will have been tested in the laboratory, increasingly in cell cultures, but also in animals in carefully controlled conditions to learn about potential side-effects. However, this is the first time the drug will have been used in patients, so no-one knows whether the new treatment will work or whether it may have unexpected risks or side-effects.

Therefore phase I trials are only offered to patients for whom no other conventional therapy remains. The primary aim is to try to find the correct dose and also the safety of the drug. The chance of an individual patient benefiting from phase I trials is very small. No more than 4% of patients actually see their tumours significantly shrink in phase I trials. You should therefore think very carefully before agreeing to such trials, which by their nature often involve frequent hospital visits and stays. They can offer hope when nothing else can usually be done, but it is more realistic to say that they are more likely to benefit other patients in the future.

Phase II trials

Phase I trials will have already shown the common side-effects, and established the correct dose of the drug. Now we need to find out whether the drug has useful anticancer effects in specific cancers. In a phase II trial, a number of patients (usually 20–50) with a specified cancer, for example advanced non-small cell lung cancer, will be treated. Usually patients will have already received and failed standard treatment. The treatment will be considered successful if some patients have tumours that shrink by at least 50% with acceptable side-effects.

Phase III trials

When a new treatment has been shown to have useful anti-cancer effects, it is now ready to be compared with existing treatments. To ensure that there is no bias in selection between the new and existing treatment, such trials are usually randomized. The treatment given is therefore allocated by chance so that at the end of the trial the treatments are balanced with patients of similar age and sex, etc., treated in each group. Only when a patient has agreed to enter the trial is the treatment selected. Neither the doctor nor patient can choose, or often actually know, which is picked—so both treatments must be acceptable to the patient. However, since both treatments are known to be effective the chances of benefit are much greater than other types of trial.

Questions about trials

Many patients understandably have concerns about being experimented on. Nowadays trials are very carefully designed, controlled and supervised to maximize patient safety. Without trials we will never know how effective treatments are, nor whether they are safer or have fewer side-effects than existing treatments. There are other benefits inasmuch as patients treated in trials may have a better outcome than those not treated in trials. This is because the treatment and follow-up is usually strictly monitored according to the trial protocol, but also because patients have access to the most up-to-date treatments.

Before any trial can start it has to be approved by the regulatory authorities within the UK, and all the documentation including patient information sheets is reviewed by an ethics committee including both lay and professional members.

All trials in the UK are run to an internationally agreed standard known as Good Clinical Practice. One important step is that patients must voluntarily sign a consent form and be fully informed about a study before any clinical trial activity can take part. These steps for research are essential for patient safety.

Before taking part in a trial you might want to ask the following questions:

- What are the possible benefits?
- What are the risks?
- How is the treatment given?
- What is known about the new treatment?
- Will it be compared with another treatment?
- If it is, will I be able to make the choice or will it be done by chance?
- Will I need to come into hospital for treatment?
- Will I need any other tests that would normally not be done?
- How long will the trial go on for?

Your team should encourage you to take part in trials. It's their way of giving you the most up-to-date treatment and trying to improve outcomes for all cancer patients.

15

Future prospects in lung cancer

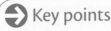 Key points

◆ Prevention by reducing smoking offers the best prospect of improving cure rates.

◆ Screening is promising using new molecular techniques.

◆ Treatment will become more individualized, dependent on the molecular make-up of each cancer.

◆ New treatments will exploit our better understanding of the biology of lung cancer.

The good news about lung cancer is that lung cancer rates are falling due to fewer people smoking. This means that in 10–20 years' time there will be 4,000–5,000 fewer people dying each year from lung cancer in developed countries. The same cannot be said of the developing world, and it is a tragedy that huge countries including India and China will have to go through the painful experiences that tobacco-related illness causes. Prevention has the highest potential to improve the dismal statistics associated with lung cancer.

Causes, risk, and prevention

We all know of people who have smoked heavily for years and don't develop lung cancer. Researchers are looking at why some smokers develop lung cancer and others do not. Normal cells become cancer cells because the genes inside them are damaged. In most cases of lung cancer, smoking causes this gene damage. If we know more about the genes that are damaged and how they are damaged, it may help in the development of new approaches to prevent the disease in the future. We look at specific genes such as *p53*, a tumour suppressor gene that specifically instructs cells to stop dividing when other genes within the DNA become damaged. The damaged cell can then undergo a process known as apoptosis, in which the cell effectively self-destructs. *p53* is either damaged or missing in most human cancers.

Other genes are also involved in the development of lung cancer, and researchers are also looking at the way in which genes may determine how tobacco smoke affects our lungs, and if our genetic make-up affects whether we want to smoke and how easy we find it to stop. Other areas of promise for the future include the study of molecular markers that help to determine risk of the disease, and chances of drugs working. In the future we hope to identify the molecular markers of a cancer and target them, both for treatment but also for improved imaging techniques and new drug delivery systems.

Chemoprevention and lung cancer
Retinoids

Chemoprevention is the use of specific natural or synthetic substances with the objective of reversing, suppressing or preventing progression to invasive cancer. Several large chemoprevention trials have been conducted, notably with retinoids. Retinoids are natural and synthetic derivatives of vitamin A. They are able to signal cells to change their genetic make-up and suppress growth effects in normal, premalignant, and malignant cells. Early work in head and neck cancer suggested that retinoids can reverse premalignant lesions and decrease the chance of developing second primary cancers. Unfortunately, when this has been tried in lung cancer patients retinoids have either shown no improvement in outcome or, worse, still more harm to those patients taking the active drug. That an apparently good idea backed up by laboratory studies can be harmful to patients is a good example of why clinical trials are essential before new treatments are introduced.

Other results support treatment with isotretinoin in 'never' and former smokers. Data from prevention trials involving selenium and vitamin E are also more encouraging for future clinical study.

Selenium

The mineral selenium has been shown in multiple studies to be an effective tool in warding off various types of cancer, including breast, oesophageal, stomach, prostate, liver, and bladder cancers. Selenium, especially when used in conjunction with vitamin C, vitamin E, and beta-carotene, works to block chemical reactions that create free radicals in the body which can damage DNA and cause degenerative change in cells, leading to cancer. Selenium also helps stop damaged DNA molecules from reproducing. In other words, selenium may act to prevent tumours from developing.

Early diagnosis and screening
Radiological tests

Screening has been shown to be successful at reducing deaths from breast, cervical and bowel cancer by detecting the disease at an earlier stage. When trials of screening chest X-rays were performed in high-risk smokers there was no improvement in survival because the disease continued to be detected in the advanced stages, even though the number of patients who could be operated upon increased.

One American trial of screening using low dose computed tomography (CT) scans has suggested that there may be some improvement in survival but this requires further confirmation. Such screening is not currently accepted practice and further large trials are planned to include many thousands of patients.

Molecular biology approaches

Another approach to lung cancer screening is to use our new knowledge of lung cancer biology as a basis for early detection. This exploits our understanding of pathways in cells whereby a cell gradually turns from being entirely normal to malignant. In other words we are hoping to detect the cancer during the process when it is starting to develop, i.e. when it is in the premalignant stages. Then, by stopping smoking and possibly by the use of other drugs as well, it may be possible to arrest or reverse the process of developing cancer. To do this, cells from either sputum samples or from biopsies taken at fibre optic bronchoscopy are analysed in the laboratory. Fluorescent bronchoscopy, which increases the sensitivity of diagnosing early cancer, has also been investigated as a possible tool for earlier diagnosis. In this method, shining different-coloured fluorescent lights onto the airway lining may help to show up abnormal cells in the airways of patients at risk of cancer, for example heavy smokers.

Other approaches are to compare blood, sputum, tissue, and urine samples from people with lung cancer and people without. If there are any differences between the two groups, particularly in the genetic structure or DNA, it might be possible to develop a straightforward test to help diagnose lung cancer.

Various molecular markers are being studied currently to detect early lung cancer. Among these, the estimation of telomerase activity holds promise as a specific marker for early, non-invasive diagnosis, as do other nuclear proteins such as A21B1, which is seen in premalignant samples taken from the lining of the airway or in sputum samples. Interestingly these proteins have been detected in sputum samples before X-rays showed a tumour.

Localized mutations in *p53* (a tumour suppressor gene) and *k-ras* genes (an oncogene) in sputum samples also appear to precede clinical symptoms or abnormal X-rays diagnostic of lung cancer. Instability within our chromosomes causing microsatellite alterations that can be detected and be markers of early cancerous change have also been reported.

There are, however, still many critical issues to be resolved in terms of molecular analysis of premalignant lesions and a proper screening programme would need to be developed and tested based on these tools.

Staging tests

We have read in Chapter 6 that it is often important to know whether or not the lymph glands in the centre of the chest are involved by tumour. Often biopsies need to be taken if there is uncertainty by mediastinoscopy (page 49) which requires an operation under general anaesthetic. New approaches not needing an operation are being developed. One method is called endobronchial ultrasound. In this method an ultrasound probe is attached to the fibre optic bronchoscope and passed into the gullet (oesophagus) and stomach, and another into the main airways and lungs. If abnormal areas in the lymph glands are found on the scan, then biopsies can be taken.

One way that treatments have improved is with better diagnostic tests. Positron emission tomography (PET) scans, for example, have reduced the number of people having surgery when the disease had already spread by about one-quarter. Such tests will not improve the results of treatment overall, but will help make the treatment more appropriate for any individual patient. For example, the tests can stop patients undergoing a major operation from which they have no chance of benefit.

Planning treatment

It seems that treatment outcomes with standard surgery, chemotherapy and radiotherapy are plateauing. Although improvements may be possible they are likely to cause a relatively small impact on the disease. The major advances are in our understanding of the biology of cancer and making our treatments more targeted. Already drugs such as bevazicumab and erlotinib are making an impact, as described in Chapter 7.

Selecting treatments: towards tailored therapy

Currently treatments are selected by the stage of the disease, histolgical type of lung cancer and the patient's fitness and wishes for treatment. For some years treatment for breast cancer has been, at least in part, tailored to the individual, initially with the identification of hormone receptors but more recently including HER2 status. (HER2 is a gene that codes a growth-promoting protein which helps control how cells divide and repair themselves. It is a poor prognostic sign in breast cancer.) At present there are no tests in lung cancer to predict whether a particular patient will or will not respond to any particular treatment. Forthcoming developments in treatment strategies for lung cancer include the use of more targeted therapies, and an ability to perform molecular assessment of individual tumours. These tumour-specific biomarkers, which are unique to an individual's cancer, will mean that the treatment can be made specific for that patient's cancer. To alter a patient's management, a biomarker needs to be predictive rather than merely prognostic. A prognostic biomarker is one where the level reflects outcome, irrespective of the treatment given. A factor is predictive if the effect of treatment is different in marker-positive or -negative patients. A marker would be useful not only if it could predict the response to treatment or likely clinical benefit, but also if it predicted no response or possibly even harm by hastening tumour progression. Any marker or test needs to be reliable, sensitive and straightforward.

Early on in their clinical use it was observed that certain factors seemed to make a response to the epidermal growth factor receptor (EGFR) inhibitors such as erlotinib more likely. Dramatic responses were observed but, importantly, not confined to females, lifelong non-smokers, adenocarcinoma histology, and those of Asian origin. Subsequently, a higher frequency of EGFR mutations was shown in these groups of patients. The aim now is to develop a test or marker of disease, such as the use of EGFR mutation identification, which can reliably predict which patients will benefit from treatment.

New treatments

Overcoming resistance to chemotherapy

A common problem with many cancers is that they become resistant to chemotherapy after one or more courses of treatment. In other words, the chemotherapy works well at first, but future courses do not help as much. Research has involved using a number of drugs such as ciclosporin to see if these agents can make resistant cells respond to chemotherapy drugs again.

Targeting altered genes

We have already seen that alterations in $p53$ may be used in early diagnosis but there is also interest in repairing or replacing abnormal $p53$ in lung cancer so that it will work normally again.

Blocking cell signals

Cells have receptors on their surfaces for a number of different proteins called growth factors. When the growth factor protein locks into its receptor on the cell surface, this tells the cell to divide into two new cells. Genes damaged within a cancer may produce too much growth factor and this acts as a signal to the other cancer cells, telling them to divide. Treatments already exist for some of these growth factors. Erlotinib targets the EGFR. Some of these proteins belong to a group called the tyrosine kinases which are discussed in Chapter 7, page 72.

Cancer vaccines

We all have vaccinations in childhood, to stop us getting certain diseases such as measles. There is already a cancer vaccine for cervical cancer. Cancer vaccines are usually designed to help treat cancer, once it has developed, by stimulating the immune system to attack the cancer cells. As yet cancer vaccines for treatment have not proved very successful because of the variability in cancer cells between different people, which means that it is difficult to develop a vaccine that can help a large number of people. However, drugs such as Stimuvax® and a vaccine called MAGE-A3 ASCI (antigen-specific cancer immunotherapeutic) are showing promise for the future. The theory is that the immune cells will then find and kill the lung cancer cells.

Blood-thinning drugs

Developing blood clots or venous thrombosis in the legs that can then spread to the lungs is a common problem for people with cancer. Lung cancer belongs to the group of malignancies with the highest incidence rates of this complication. The overall risk of venous thrombosis was found to be increased seven-fold in patients with cancer compared to those without. Cancer treatments, particularly chemotherapy, can also increase the risk of blood clots. The risk of venous thrombosis is highest in the first few months after the diagnosis of malignancy and when the cancer has spread. It seems that people with lung cancer who take warfarin, a blood-thinning drug, may live longer than those who don't take it. However, this only works for those people in whom the cancer has spread. Unfortunately the level of warfarin is difficult to control in cancer patients, and there is a major risk of bleeding; it is not clear if the possible benefits of taking warfarin outweighs this risk. Trials are ongoing with more modern, safer, blood-thinning drugs. Interestingly some doctors believe that blood-thinning treatments may also reduce the spread of cancer cells.

The future

The key remains prevention and then earlier diagnosis of this illness. New treatment strategies are more likely to control rather than eradicate the disease.

Appendix

Sources of help, information, and advice

The internet is a seemingly unlimited source of daily information. Googling 'lung cancer' will get you 17,900,000 references. Although there is no shortage of information, it is important to remember that anyone can post whatever they like on the internet, whether it be true or not.

The Roy Castle Lung Cancer Foundation is the only charity in the UK wholly dedicated to defeating lung cancer:

http://www.roycastle.org/

Two other good starts with reliable links are the Cancer Research UK website (CRUK):

http://www.cancerresearchuk.org/

and Cancerbackup site, now part of Macmillan Cancer Support:

http://www.cancerbackup.org.uk/Cancertype/Lung

Other reputable and useful sites include the British Lung Foundation:

http://www.lunguk.org/you-and-your-lungs/conditions-and-diseases/lung-cancer.htm

Increasingly in the UK the National Institute for Health and Clinical Excellence makes recommendations not only about individual treatments but also about the overall management of conditions:

http://www.nice.org.uk/

http://www.nice.org.uk/CG024

Similar guidelines exist in Wales:

http://www.wales.nhs.uk/sites3/documents/362/Lung_Eng.pdf

and Scotland:

http://www.sign.ac.uk/pdf/sign80.pdf

It's bad enough having a diagnosis of cancer. This review by the National Cancer Institute of America is helpfully entitled 'Facing Forward: Life After Cancer Treatment'. It is a guide of what to do after cancer:

http://www.cancer.gov/cancertopics/life-after-treatment/page1

Here is a calculator to work out how many cigarettes you have smoked, otherwise known as tobacco pack-years:

http://www.smokingpackyears.com/

Glossary

Acquired immunodeficiency syndrome (AIDS): illness resulting from human immunodeficiency virus (HIV).

Acupuncture: A method of healing developed in China at least 2,000 years ago, for the treatment of pain or disease by inserting the tips of needles at specific points on the skin.

Adenoma: a benign tumour arising from glands.

Adenocarcinoma: tumour of the glands.

Adjuvant: usually treatment as a follow-up to surgery designed to remove any microscopic traces of tumour which may be left behind.

Adrenal glands: glands that sit on top of the kidney that secrete hormones.

Adrenocorticotrophic hormone (ACTH): stimulates the production of hormones from the adrenal gland.

Anaemia: lack of red blood cells.

Angiogenesis: growth of new blood vessels.

Antibody: substance produced by the body to fight infection.

Aspirate: to withdraw fluid.

Aspirin: a common pain-killer.

Biopsy: removal of tissue or fluid for examination under a microscope.

Bronchi: the trachea divides into two tubes (the bronchi). One goes into each lung.

Bronchitis: inflammation of the bronchi.

Bronchoscope: an instrument inserted down the trachea so that the doctor can see inside the bronchi.

Bronchoscopy: the technique of using a bronchoscope.

Cancer: a general term for growths in the body. Cancers tend to cause destruction of nearby tissues, spread to other parts of the body, and can recur after removal.

Cancer *in situ*: a small tumour that has not spread from its original site.

Carcinogen: a substance that promotes cancer.

Carcinoma: a malignant growth of epithelial tissue like the skin and glands.

Chemotherapy: treatment using drugs.

Chromosome: the genetic material found in every cell in the body. Every human cell contains 46 chromosomes, which carry the genes.

Combination chemotherapy: treatment with a combination of drugs.

Corticosteroid: steroid hormones produced by the adrenal glands.

Cryotherapy: freezing tumours.

Cytology: examination of individual cells under the microscope.

DNA: our genetic structure.

Dose–response effect: the effect of different doses on the response to a treatment.

Dysplasia: development of abnormal tissue.

Electron microscope: a very high resolution microscope.

Emphysema: damage to the lungs caused by loss of fine air pockets (alveoli).

Endobronchial: refers to the lining of the airway.

Excision: removal by cutting out.

Gene: a chemical structure on the chromosome that is responsible for passing on hereditary information.

Haemoptysis: coughing up blood.

Hormone: a chemical secreted into the bloodstream that controls the functioning of the rest of the body.

Human immunodeficiency virus (HIV): infection with the virus may result in acquired immunodeficiency syndrome (AIDS).

Hyperthermia: heating to achieve a very high body temperature.

Immunotherapy: treatment that uses the body's immune system to fight the cancer.

Inflammation: reaction of tissues to infection. Characterized by pain, swelling, redness, and heat.

Isotope: a chemical that can exist in two physical forms. Radioactive isotopes are used in medical research because their position can be monitored.

Large cell cancer: type of cancer found in smokers. May develop in the central or peripheral parts of the lungs. Can spread to the airways, lymph glands, and to other parts of the body in the bloodstream.

Larynx: the voice box.

Laser: 'Light Amplification by Stimulated Emission of Radiation'. Energy transmitted as heat that can destroy cells.

Latent period: period between exposure to a carcinogen and development of cancer.

Lobectomy: excision of a lobe.

Localized disease: disease confined to one part of the body.

Lymph glands: filter lymph fluid and make up part of the lymphatic system involved in removing bacteria. An important part of the immune system.

Magnetic resonance imaging (MRI): a type of scan that does not use X-rays.

Malaise: feeling tired and unwell.

Malignant: dangerous, fatal.

Mediastinum: the area in the middle of the chest containing the heart, great vessels, oesophagus, and other structures.

Mesothelioma: tumour of the lining of the lung. It is associated with exposure to asbestos.

Metaplasia: transformation of one type of cell into a different type.

Metastasis: the transference or spread of disease from one part of the body to another.

Metastasize: the process of metastasis.

Metastatic: a tumour that has the ability to metastasize.

Monoclonal antibody: strain of antibody that can be used to differentiate tumours.

Mortality: the death rate.

Mucosa: a membrane/lining that contains glands.

Nausea: sickness.

Neutropenia: low white blood cell count.

Oedema: swelling of tissue caused by fluid.

Oesophagus: the gullet.

Oncogene: gene capable of stimulating the formation of a tumour.

Paraneoplastic: disease associated with malignancy but that is not directly caused by the tumour.

Paroxysm: a sudden attack.

Passive smoking: inhalation of other people's cigarette smoke.

Pathology: examination of specimens under the microscope.

Pericardial: referring to the sac that surrounds the heart.

Photodynamic therapy (PDT): uses light-activated drugs.

Phototherapy: treatment by exposure to artificial blue light.

Placebo: a harmless, inert substance that looks identical to the substance being tested.

Pleura: membrane lining the lungs.

Pleural effusion: fluid in the space between the lung and the chest wall.

Pleuritic pain: pain in the lining of the lungs.

Pneumonectomy: removal of a lung.

Positron emission tomography (PET): a type of body scan that measures activity which tends to be higher in a tumour.

Precancerous: changes that occur before a cancer forms. They usually result in cancer.

Prophylactic: preventive.

Radiotherapy: treatment by X-rays.

Remission: period when the cancer has reduced in size or disappeared.

Resection: surgical removal (excision).

Sarcoma: malignant growth of bone and muscle.

Secondary tumour: metastasis of a tumour from another part of the body.

Squamous cell lung cancer: common in smokers. Cancerous cells develop in the airways.

Steroid: naturally occurring group of hormones.

Thoracotomy: surgical exposure of the chest cavity.

TNM system (tumour, node, metastasis): international system of staging cancers.

Trachea: the windpipe.

Tumour: mass of abnormal tissue that resembles normal tissue but that serves no useful purpose. May be benign (does not infiltrate nearby tissue or cause metastases; unlikely to recur if removed) or malignant.

Ultrasound: a technique for visualizing inner structures of the body by analysing the echoes of very high-pitched sound.

Index

regional nodes 46
relapse, treatment at 76
simplified staging system 44–5
small molecule technology 72
stages 74–6
surgery 44, 47, 59–64, 74–5
targeted therapies 71–4
tests used to stage lung cancer 44–7
TNM system 44
treatment 59–74
non-surgical treatment 64–71
North America, smoking in 10, 17
Northern Ireland, smoking in 20
nurses 57–8, 73, 112

occupational exposure 12–13, 22, 86
occurrence of lung cancer 4–6
oedema 101
oils 12
oncologists 113
operations *see* **surgery**
organization of services,
  improvements in 80
organizations
  Action on Smoking and Health (ASH) 32
  British Lung Foundation 133
  Cancer Research UK 133
  Cancerbackup 133
  QUIT charity 28, 32
  Roy Castle Lung Cancer Foundation
    118, 133
  stopping smoking 28, 32
  support organizations 118
osteoarthropathy 39
osteoporosis 100
Our Healthier Nation **strategy** 111
outpatient treatment 70
oxycodone 105

packaging, health warnings on 23
pack-years 19, 134
Paclitaxel 70
pain
  acupuncture 106
  addiction 104
  anaesthetic, injections of local 105–6
  aspirin 104
  bones, spread to the 99–100
  buprenorphine 105
  chemotherapy 103

chest pain 37–8, 67, 84
chronic pain 104
codeine 104
complications, treatment of 103–6
constipation 104, 105
depression and stress 104, 105, 107
dosage 105
drugs 103–5
fentanyl patches 105
hypnosis 106
laxatives 105
mesothelioma 84
mild pain 104
moderate pain 104–5
morphine 104, 105
nerve blocks 105–6
night, worsening at 103–4
oxycodone 105
painkillers 61, 62, 100, 103–5
paracetamol 104
radiotherapy 103
severe pain 105
side-effects of painkillers 100, 104, 105
surgery 61, 62
swallowing, pain on 66
symptoms, treatment of 103–6
tiredness 105
transcutaneous nerve stimulation
  (TNS) 106
WHO ladder for painkillers 104
palliative treatment 57, 64, 67, 76, 80,
  84–6, 113–14
pamidronate 98
pancoast tumours 53
paracemator 104
paraneoplastic phenomena 102
paraneoplastic syndromes 38–9
partners of patients 122
passive smoking 20–21, 25, 34
pastoral care workers 113
pathologists 112
peer pressure and smoking 32, 33
peer review 111
pemetrexed 70, 86
percutaneous radiofrequency
  ablation 91
performance status 54–5, 80
pericardial effusion 96–7
peritoneum 82–3
petroleum products and oils 12